D0043393

FANGCANG SHELTER HOSPITALS FOR COVID-19

CONSTRUCTION AND OPERATION MANUAL

FANGCANG SHELTER HOSPITALS FOR COVID-19

CONSTRUCTION AND OPERATION MANUAL

Editior-in-Chief
Yan Zhi

Translator
Yan Ge

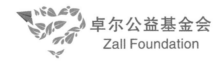

卓尔公益基金会
Zall Foundation

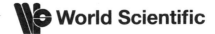

NEW JERSEY · LONDON · SINGAPORE · BEIJING · SHANGHAI · HONG KONG · TAIPEI · CHENNAI · TOKYO

Published by

World Scientific Publishing Co. Pte. Ltd.
5 Toh Tuck Link, Singapore 596224
USA office: 27 Warren Street, Suite 401-402, Hackensack, NJ 07601
UK office: 57 Shelton Street, Covent Garden, London WC2H 9HE

British Library Cataloguing-in-Publication Data
A catalogue record for this book is available from the British Library.

FANGCANG SHELTER HOSPITALS FOR COVID-19
Construction and Operation Manual

Copyright © Zall Foundation, 2020

All rights reserved.

ISBN 978-981-122-306-8 (hardcover)
ISBN 978-981-122-307-5 (paperback)
ISBN 978-981-122-308-2 (ebook for institutions)
ISBN 978-981-122-309-9 (ebook for individuals)

To learn more about this book, please visit
https://www.worldscientific.com/worldscibooks/10.1142/11904

Desk Editor: Tan Boon Hui

Typeset by Art Department

Contents

Foreword

The novel coronavirus (SARS-CoV-2) is a newly emerging pathogen, and has the characteristics of strong infectivity and fast propagation. The transmission of the SARS-CoV-2 occurs through respiratory droplets between people with close contact. China and other countries have identified and reported coronavirus disease 2019 (COVID-19) cases.

As a novel public health concept, the Fangcang Shelter Hospital was first proposed in February 2020, in Wuhan, China, by Professor Wang Chen, an academician of Chinese Academy Engineering. While responding to the coronavirus disease 2019 (COVID-19) outbreak, medical staff faced the pressing situation of limited medical supplies, which led Professor Wang Chen to the suggestion of converting large-scale public venues such as exhibition centers and indoor stadiums into shelter hospitals to receive large numbers of patients, as this involved minimum time and monetary cost. The five essential functions of Fangcang Shelter Hospitals, namely isolation, triage, basic medical care, close monitoring and rapid referral, and essential living and social engagement enable shelter hospitals to receive patients with mild to moderate symptoms of COVID-19, and have the greatest impact on isolating the source of infection and expanding the area's healthcare capacity.

With the great experience from Zall Foundation's crews who contributed to the design, renovation and operation of these shelter hospitals, this booklet encompasses knowledge and experience distilled from the running of these Fangcang Shelter Hospitals. Covering five important aspects, including the proposal, design, renovation, operation and logistical support for shelter hospitals, this manual aims to be a useful reference for other epidemic prevention and control work in regions around the world.

Yan Zhi
Founder of Zall Foundation
April 2020

Chapter 1

Proposing Strategies of Establishment of Fangcang Shelter Hospital

1.1 Construction Background of Fangcang Shelter Hospital

Wuhan, a metropolitan city with millions of people, went into lockdown on January 23, 2020, to interrupt the transmission of the novel coronavirus. The number of confirmed cases of COVID-19 grew rapidly, which overburdened medical resources. The situation of "A ward bed is hard to beg for" emerged. In this case, a large number of confirmed patients could not be admitted to the hospital and had to choose home quarantine. Prof. Wang Chen, Vice President of Chinese Academy of Engineering, President of Chinese Academy of Medical Sciences, and an expert in Pulmonary and Critical Care Medicine (PC-CM) supported at the front line in the fight against the epidemic. He put forward the idea of constructing Fangcang Shelter Hospital as soon as possible, on January 1, after full investigation, to implement the strategy of "All suspected and confirmed patients should be admitted to the hospital and all confirmed patients should be treated". The China Culture Expo Center of Wuhan Salon, Wuhan

International Conference and Exhibition Center, and Hongshan Gymnasium in Wuhan were expropriated on February 3, to build the first batches of Fangcang Shelter Hospitals in Wuhan.

Fangcang Shelter Hospital was constructed using mainly existing buildings or resources, to admit COVID-19 patients with mild to moderate symptoms in the shortest time and at minimum cost, to the greatest extent. This not only provides basic medical care for patients, transfers them to designated hospitals and provides them with basic living conditions, but also controls the source of infection effectively and cuts off the route of transmission of the virus, which prevents the spread of pandemic, improves the recovery rate and reduces the fatality rate. The construction of Fangcang Shelter Hospital is not a "perfect strategy", but an advisable and realistic strategy. In the course of epidemic prevention and control in China, Fangcang Shelter Hospital plays an important role, which provides a new idea and creates a new model for other countries in dealing with the epidemic and expanding medical resources rapidly.

The number of confirmed cases of COVID-19 is on the rise all over the world, which results in a desperate lack of medical resources in all countries, especially the number of ward beds for the treatment of confirmed patients. A significant proportion of confirmed patients cannot be admitted to the hospital and receive treatment under quarantine. Self-quarantine at home will put family members at risk, cause cross infection and lead to further spread of the epidemic.

Upon the establishment of Fangcang Shelter Hospital, scientific classification and treatment measures can be adopted, to admit severe patients and critical patients into designated hospitals. A large number of patients with mild to moderate symptoms are admitted into Fangcang Shelter Hospital in a centralized way, which improves the utilization efficiency of medical resources.

1.2 Definition of Fangcang Shelter Hospital

Fangcang Shelter Hospital in China is a large improvised hospital which is constructed rapidly by reconstructing the convention and exhibition centers, stadiums and other existing large places into medical facilities. It is used to isolate a large number of COVID-19 patients with mild to moderate symptoms from family members and communities, and also provide medical care, disease surveillance and referral as well as living and social spaces.

1.3 Characteristics of Fangcang Shelter Hospital

An article "Fangcang Shelter Hospital: A New Idea for Responding to Public Health Emergencies" focusing on China's construction and use of Fangcang Shelter Hospitals was published on April 2 in *The Lancet,* one of the world's top medical journals. This article was prepared jointly by Prof. Wang Chen and the Heidelberg Institute of Global Health, at the University of Heidelberg, Germany. Three characteristics of Fangcang Shelter Hospital are listed in the article:

fast construction, large scale and low cost. These characteristics enable it to respond to public health emergencies in an efficient way.

Patients unable to be admitted to hospitals are mainly admitted to Fangcang Shelter Hospital, which not only prevents infection to family members but also provides timely medical treatment for the patients. All patients admitted to Fangcang Shelter Hospital are those tested positive in the nucleic acid testing (NAT) which rules out infection factors of influenza. Admitted patients should wear masks and other preventive measures are also taken. Therefore, there is basically no cross infection between patients admitted into Fangcang Shelter Hospital.

1.4 Functions of Fangcang Shelter Hospital

The Fangcang Shelter hospital has five essential functions:

(1) Isolation. For patients with mild to moderate symptoms, it has better effect than self-quarantine at home.

(2) Triage. It provides a strategic function for confirmed COVID-19 patients. Mild to moderate COVID-19 patients are admitted to Fangcang Shelter Hospital for treatment in isolation, while severe and critical COVID-19 patients are treated in normal hospitals, thus effectively releasing capacity pressure of the local hospitals.

(3) Provision of basic medical care. This includes antiviral, antipyretic and antibiotic treatment, support of oxygen and

intravenous fluids, and mental health counseling.

(4) Frequent monitoring and rapid referral. The patient's conditions such as breathing frequency, body temperature, oxygen saturation are measured frequently every day. The patients who meet certain clinical criteria are quickly transferred to designated higher-level medical institutions for treatment. This greatly reduces referral time before the patients' conditions worsen.

(5) Provision of a community for patients, with living essentials and social engagement. Fangcang Shelter Hospital provides a community for patients with mild symptoms to moderate symptoms, where there are mutual assistance between the medical staff and patients, and social activities participated by the patients will ease the anxiety caused by the disease and isolation, so as to promote rehabilitation.

Chapter 2

Fangcang Shelter Hospitals Project Design

2.1 Function Division

Fangcang Shelter Hospitals should be designed under the principle of "Three zones, two passages"; this means the traffic should be organized in a way where medical staff and patients can be separated, while contaminated passages and clean passages are separated. The negative pressure ventilation system should be installed. Moreover, there should be enough space for living and social engagement.

The three zones are namely: contaminated zone, semi-contaminated zone and clean zone. Clean zone: for medical staff who have low risk of exposing to patients' blood, body fluids, pathogenic microorganisms and other polluted or infected materials. Confirmed patients with infectious disease are prohibited from entering the area. Semi-contaminated zone: located between contaminated zone and clean zone, for medical staff who have medium risk of exposing to patients' blood, body fluids, pathogenic microorganisms and other contaminated or infected materials. Contaminated zone: where suspected and confirmed patients with infectious disease are being treated and cured. Blood, body fluids, secretion, medical waste and any contaminated materials are disposed in this area. There should be a clear and obvious sign to distinct different areas, and isolation belts can also be used. The areas can be differentiated by colored signs. "Two passages" are namely health workers' passage and patients' passage. Moreover, cleansing passage and contaminated zone should be strictly separated to avoid any unnecessary interactions between medical staff and patients.

When passing through contaminated zone from clean zone, the entrance used should be labeled as "sanitary entering room" and "sanitary exit room".

The entering procedure should be: first changing room — second changing room — buffer room. After all protective equipment are donned, the medical staff can approach the contaminated zone.

The returning procedure should be: buffer room — isolation suits taken off — buffer room — showering — changing room, after which, one may proceed to the clean zone. The sanitary exit room should be distinguished by gender.

2.2 Ward Bed Area Design

The bed area should be divided into male section and female section. Every bed area should be allocated with no more than 42 beds. There should be 2 exits, located within 30m away from any point of the bed area. The corridor between two different areas should be used as evacuation corridors. In a large, open space area, the width of the evacuation corridor should be no less than 4m. The evacuation corridor should be indicated with clear signs. The material used for isolation belt located between different bed area should be incombustible or flame retardant. The surface of the belt should be scrub resistant, while the height of the belt should not be lower than 1.8m. Beds shall be arranged with proper spacing, and comfortable enough for treatment and monitoring. The distance between two parallel beds should be no less than 1.4m. When placing beds in a single line, the distance between bed and the wall opposite should be no less then 1.1m.

2.3 Toilet Design

The toilets for medical and patients should be set up separately. The toilets for patients should be temporary, and a special passage should be set between the temporary toilet and the ward area. Foam-blocked portable toilets should be used if it is possible. The number of toilet and population ratio should be 1:20 for male, and 1:10 for female. The number of toilets can be adjusted according to reasonable needs and requirements from patients. Polluted water from toilet should be first discharged to specialized tanks for disinfection, before distributing into urban sewerage and drainage pipes.

The existing toilets in the public venue can be provided for medical staff and logistics support staff who are in healthy conditions. Toilets can be closed if it is not in use.

2.4 Firefighting and Barrier Free Design

The admission capacity should be determined based on the width of emergency exit and evacuation stairs. The evacuation space should be able to contain 100 people or designed according to relevant fire prevention regulations.

The main entrance and exit, as well as all the channels to different departments, should be provided with barrier free corridors. There should be rampway design when there is a height difference; the falling gradient should strictly follow the relevant constriction code. The width of the barrier free corridor should be large enough to contain both wheelchair patients and the caregivers.

2.5 Design of Auxiliary Rooms

There should be a specific locker room for personal belongings, a disinfection and security check room, and patients changing room located in the entrance. When transferring or discharging patients, there should be an area for packing and disinfection. Moreover, the location of emergency resuscitation room, diet preparation room, equipment storage, filth cleaning room, and daily garbage storage should be near the bed area. The pharmacy, medical equipment storage, medicine storage, diet preparation room, duty room and office should be located near the medical staff working area.

2.6 Fangcang Shelter Hospitals Design Case Reference

In a city with high population density, public venues such as indoor stadiums, exhibition centers, departure halls, factories, school function halls, can be redeveloped into Fangcang Shelter Hospitals. Some reference cases are shown as below.

2.6.1 Single-floor Exhibition Center Fangcang Shelter Hospital

Reference case: we took Wuhan Salon: Cultural Exhibition Center under Zall Property as an example which was redeveloped into a single-floor Fangcang Shelter Hospital in the East-West Lake District. Zall (Wuhan Salon) Fangcang Shelter Hospital was reconstructed on the base of three exhibition hall (Hall A, B and C). The detailed layout is shown in Fig. 2-2.

We first studied and evaluated the original layout and construction drawing of the exhibition center, then carried out a site investigation. Based on these information and investigation results, as well as the relevant regulation and standards, our experts formulated an achievable construction plan.

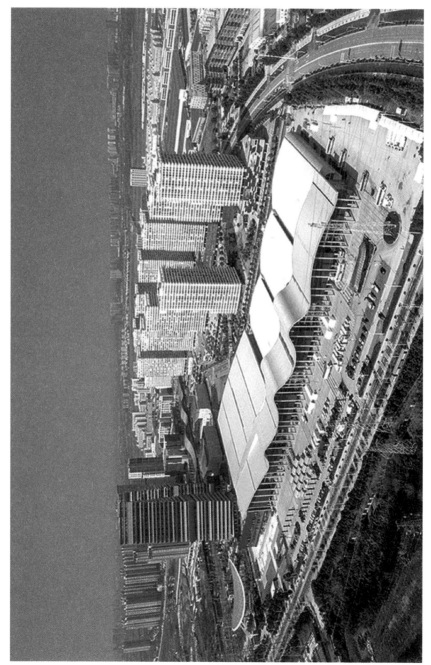

Fig. 2-1 Aerial View of Zall (Wuhan Salon) Fangcang Shelter Hospital

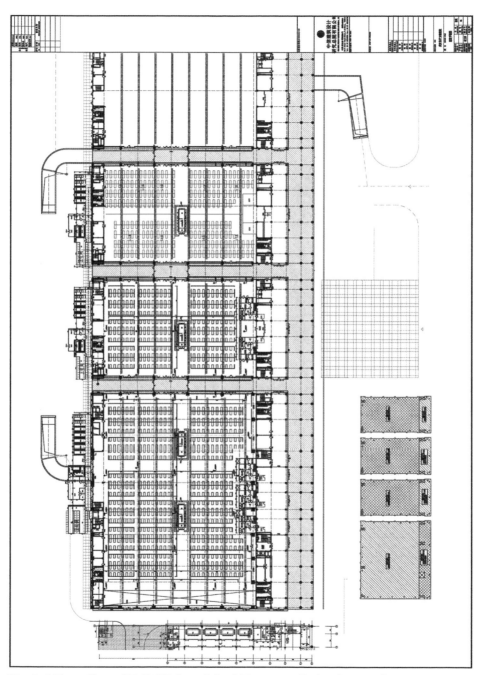

Fig. 2-2 Floor Plan of Zall (Wuhan Salon) Fangcang Shelter Hospital

Zall (Wuhan Salon) Fangcang Shelter Hospital is divided into "three zones and two passages" (see Fig. 2-2), and reconstruction plan was designed according to the function requirements of professional hospitals, to admit and treat patients. Functional renovation is carried out for the main exhibition hall (Exhibition Hall A) and two side exhibition halls (Exhibition Hall B and Hall C) according to the plan of Wuhan Salon's Chinese Cultural Exhibition Center. The contaminated zone is used for medical treatment and admission of patients; the clean zone is for living engagement and supplies; the halls in between are used as an area for sanitary passages. The medical staff dormitory is located near the hospital. They are allowed to return home after 14-days quarantine in the medical staff dormitory.

Key point 1: We can take advantage of the large space in the exhibition hall, to allocate wards and medical working areas, which are separated and designed in a fishbone layout. The medical working area is located in the center, with wards on both sides of working area, which are directly connected with it. Once the hospital receive a patient on the peripheral side, the basic treatment procedures are: admitted from patient's passage in lateral side — treatment completed — disinfected in clean zone — discharged.

Key point 2: Areas for living engagement and medical and living supplies should be provided. The space around the existing entrance for supplies are used as storage for urgent medical supplies.

There should also be an independent entrance and exit for medical staff, and set up of on-call rooms, offices, consultation rooms and telemedicine rooms nearby. There should be a sanitary room connected to the medical working area. The detailed plan is shown in Fig. 2-6.

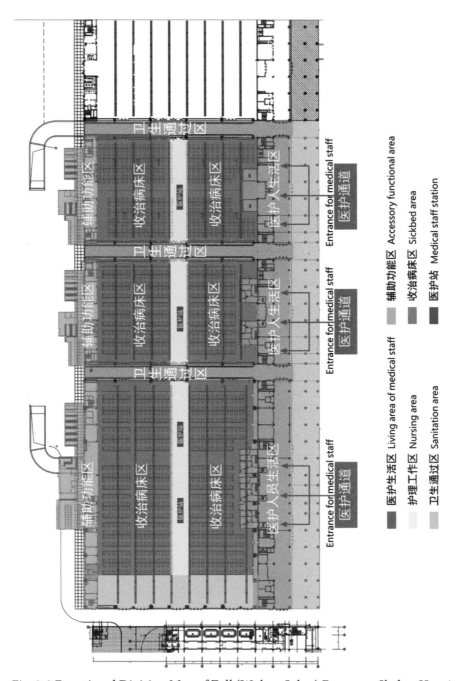

Fig. 2-3 Functional Division Map of Zall (Wuhan Salon) Fangcang Shelter Hospital

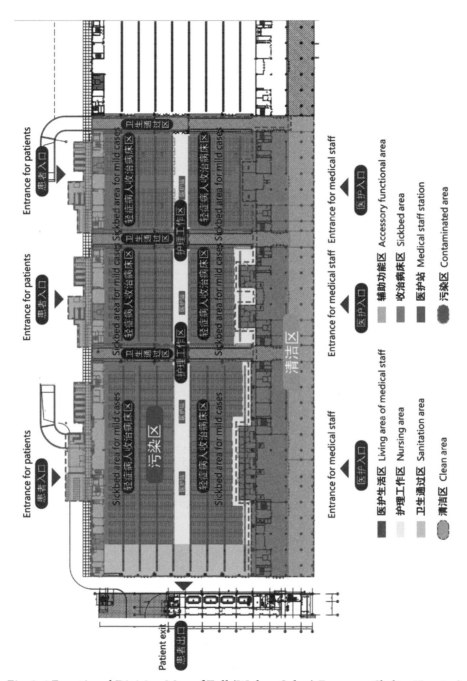

Fig. 2-4 Functional Division Map of Zall (Wuhan Salon) Fangcang Shelter Hospital

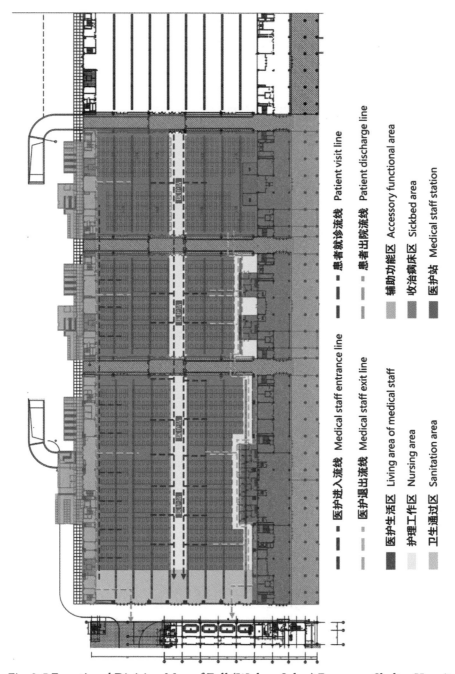

Fig. 2-5 Functional Division Map of Zall (Wuhan Salon) Fangcang Shelter Hospital

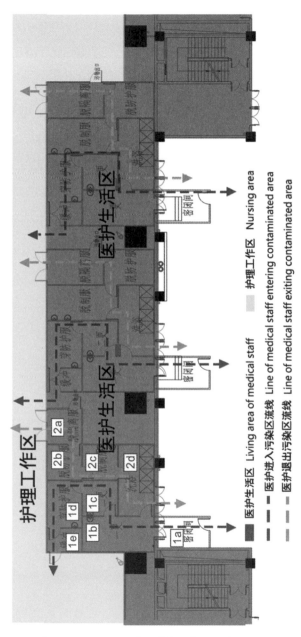

Fig. 2-6 Functional Division Map of Zall (Wuhan Salon) Fangcang Shelter Hospital

2.6.2 Multi-Floor Exhibition Center Fangcang Shelter Hospital

Reference Case: We can use Zall (Jianghan, Wuzhan) Fangcang Shelter Hospital reconstructed from Wuhan International Exhibition Center in Jianghan District as an example for Multi-floor Exhibition Center Fangcang Shelter Hospital. Just like Zall (Wuhan Salon) Fangcang Shelter Hospital, it is reconstructed based on a large space exhibition hall, except that Zall (Jianghan Wuzhan) Fangcang Shelter Hospital has two floors. The first floor is clean area or semi-polluted clean area, while second floor is polluted and contaminated area. Detailed plan is shown in Fig. 2-7 and Fig. 2-8.

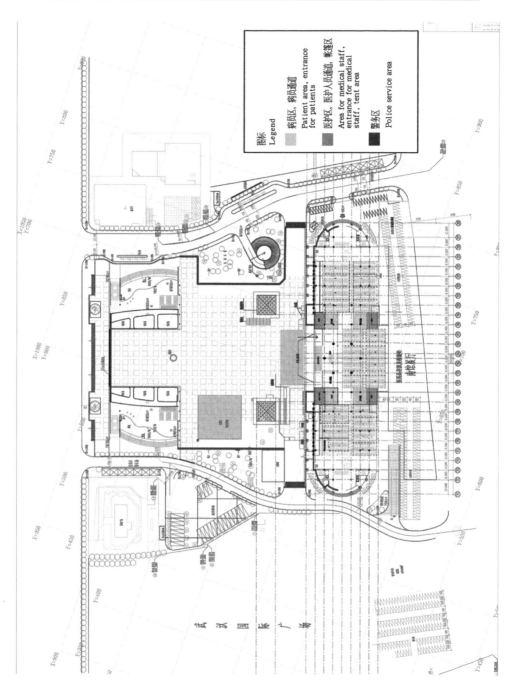

Fig. 2-7 Plan of Zall (Jianghan Wuzhan) Fangcang Shelter Hospital First Floor

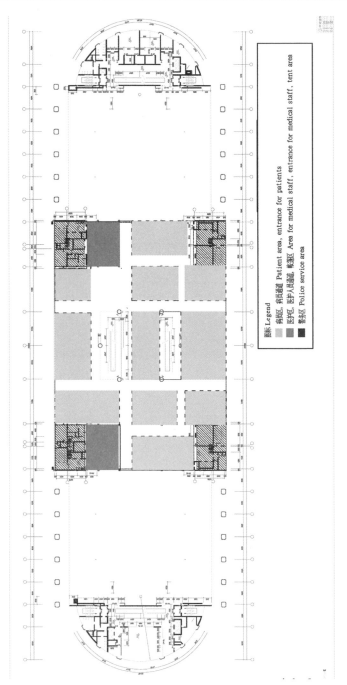

Fig. 2-8 Plan of Zall (Jianghan Wuzhan) Fangcang Shelter Hospital Second Floor

2.6.3 Indoor Stadium Fangcang Shelter Hospital

Reference Case: Wuchang Fangcang Shelter Hospital. It was reconstructed from Hongshan Indoor Stadium in Wuchang, Wuhan, and redeveloped based on an indoor basketball court. The construction drawings are shown in Fig. 2-9 to 2-14.

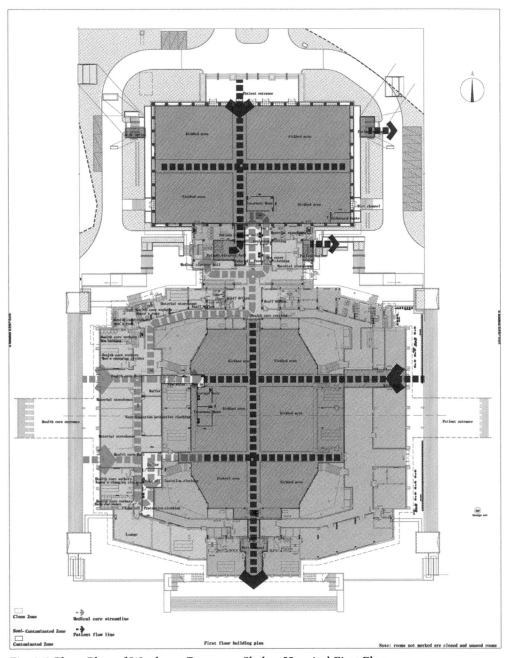

Fig. 2-9 Floor Plan of Wuchang Fangcang Shelter Hospital First Floor

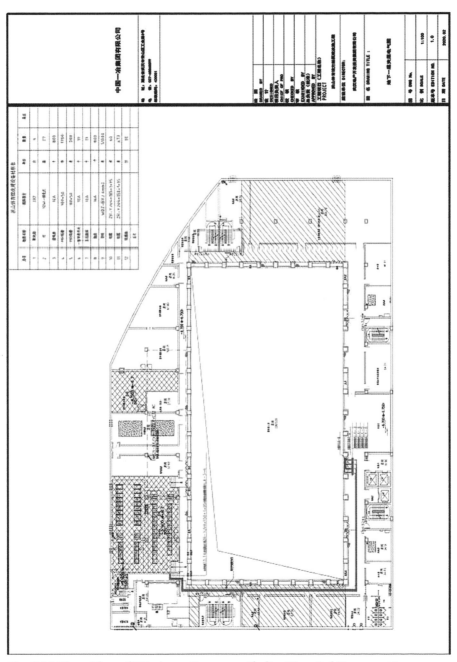

Fig. 2-10 Floor Plan of Wuchang Fangcang Shelter Hospital Basement 1

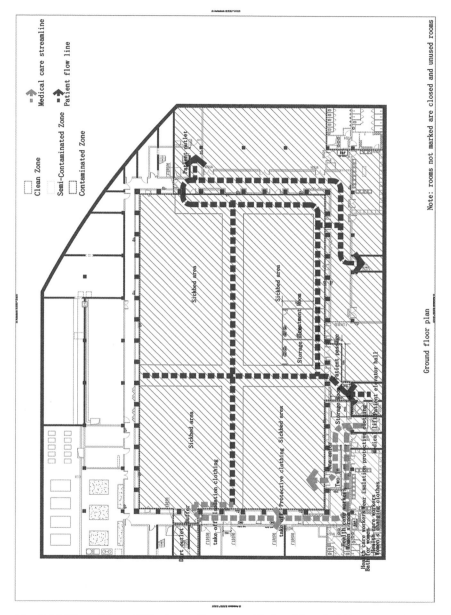

Fig. 2-11 Floor Plan of Wuchang Fangcang Shelter Hospital Basement 1

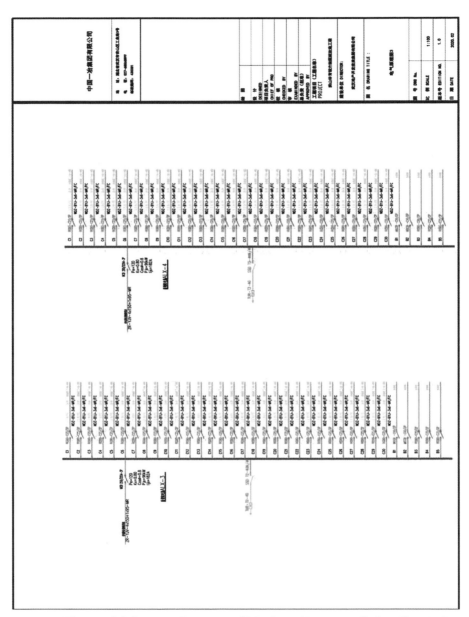

Fig. 2-12 Electrical Schematic Diagram of Wuchang Fangcang Shelter Hospital

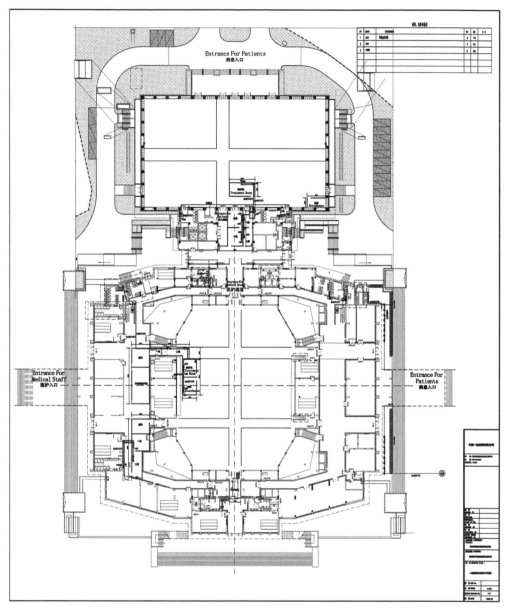

Fig. 2-13 Building, Water Supply and Drainage Plan of Wuchang Fangcang Shelter Hospital
First Floor

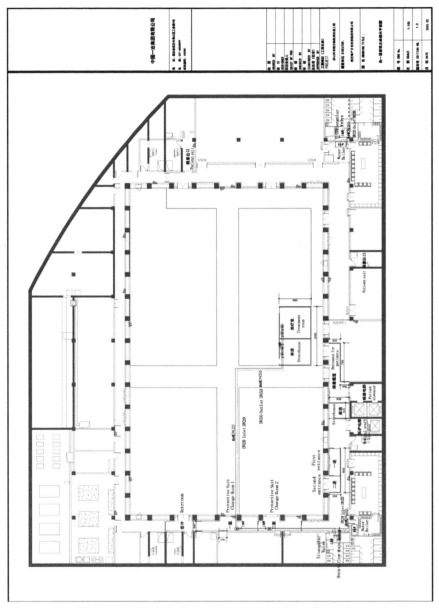

Fig. 2-14 Building, Water Supply and Drainage Plan of Wuchang Fangcang Shelter Hospital Basement 1

2.6.4 Vacant Factory Fangcang Shelter Hospital

Reference Case: Zall Rehabilitation Station in Changjiang New Town, Wuhan. This Fangcang Shelter Hospital is a combination of 10 small "shelter rooms", the surface area of each shelter room is 12000m^2. The detailed plan is shown in Fig. 2-15.

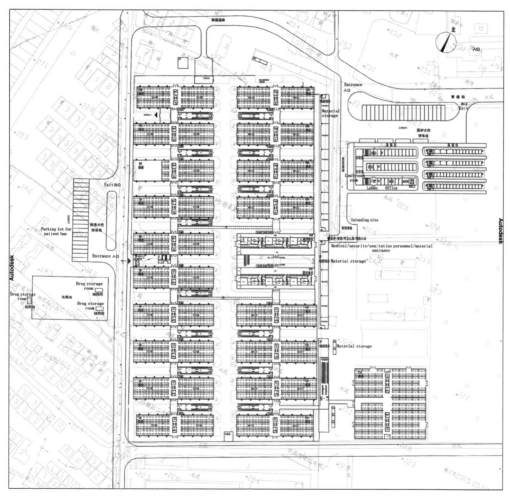

Fig. 2-15 Floor Plan of Zall Rehabilitation Station in Changjiang New Town

2.6.5 Departure Hall Fangcang Shelter Hospital

Reference Case: Zall (Hankou North) Fangcang Shelter Hospital. It was reconstructed based on a departure hall in a train station. It is located in Hankou North Passenger Terminal in Huangpi District, Wuhan. The detailed layout plan is shown in Fig. 2-16.

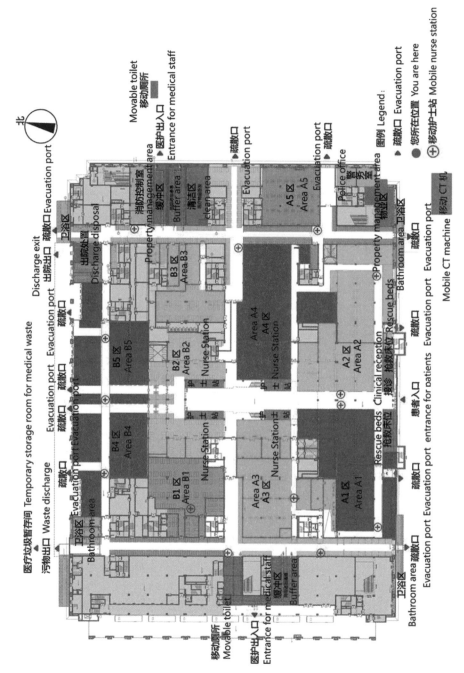

Fig. 2-16 Zoning Plan of Zall (North Hankou) Fangcang Shelter Hospital

2.6.6 Multifunction School Venue Fangcang Shelter Hospital

Reference case: Hanyang Fangcang Shelter Hospital in Hanyang District, Wuhan. It was reconstructed based on a three-floor multi-function sports hall (surface area: 13000 m²) and a tennis court (4800m²) in Sports School, Wuhan. The detailed layout plan is shown in Fig. 2-17 to 2-20.

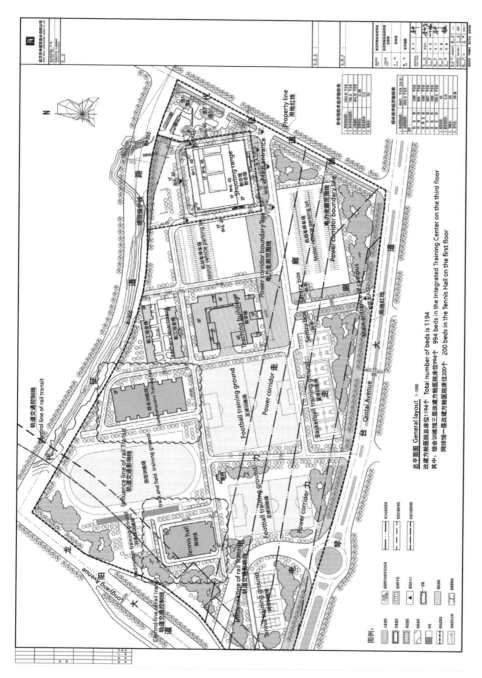

Fig. 2-17 Floor Plan of Hanyang Fangcang Shelter Hospital

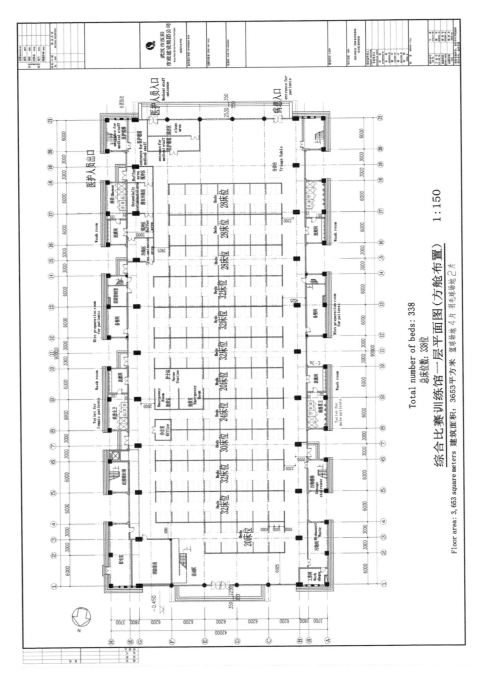

Fig. 2-18 Floor Plan of Hanyang Fangcang Shelter Hospital First Floor

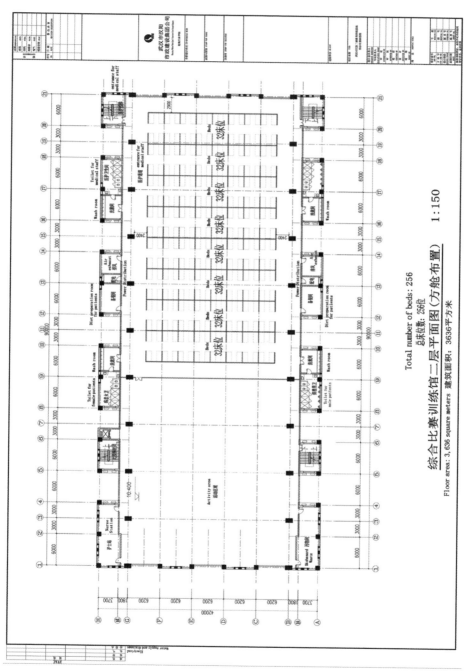

Fig. 2-19 Floor Plan of Hanyang Fangcang Shelter Hospital Second Floor

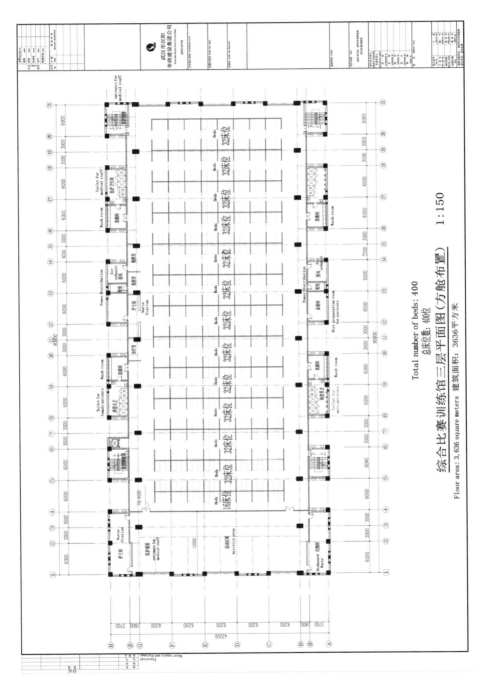

Fig. 2-20 Floor Plan of Hanyang Fangcang Shelter Hospital Third Floor

Chapter 3

Fangcang Shelter Hospitals Reconstruction

3.1 Content of Reconstruction

3.1.1 The Reconstruction Principles

The reconstruction process of Fangcang Shelter Hospitals involves the following aspects: infrastructure provided by local government, sewage treatment facility, internal separation belt construction, indoor equipment and facilities, circulation routes to outside traffic, supplies transportation corridors, neighborhood environment design and construction; epidemic prevention and control facilities, biological safety facilities and security.

Until the end of expropriation period, the public venues can be solely used as Fangcang Shelter Hospitals, for receiving and treating the suspected and confirmed COVID-19 patients.

The reconstruction of the existing property must strictly comply with the relevant epidemic prevention and control regulations and infectious diseases hospitals' standards.

If the relevant regulations and standards cannot be met, reasonable adjustments on the property reconstruction plan should be made based on the actual situation.

3.1.2 Reference Cases

Venues such as exhibition halls, indoor stadiums, train station departure halls, multi-function sports halls and vacant factories should be renovated in the following aspects: sewage system, ventilation system, power system and ward areas, in order to redevelop into a Fangcang Shelter Hospital. We now study Zall (Wuhan Salon) Fangcang Shelter Hospital and use it as a reference case for Fangcang Shelter Hospitals reconstruction project.

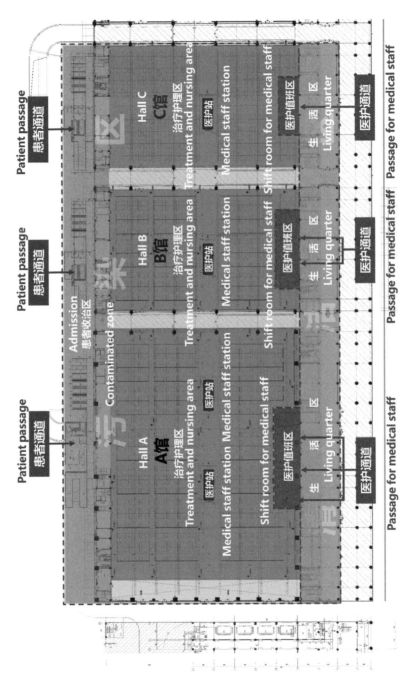

Fig. 3-1 Floor Plan of Zall (Wuhan Salon) Fangcang Shelter Hospital

(1) Install strong electricity wire in Hall A, B and C. Each hall should be allocated with approximately 1500 beds. Sockets should be installed next to bed in every ward. For security purpose, there should be an interior partition device set up in the hall.

(2) Power system should be installed in nurse station, medical waste room, storage room, and treatment room in Hall A, B and C.

(3) Mechanical air supply and air exhaust systems in semi-contaminated areas (first changing room, second changing room, buffer room, room for donning/doffing personal protective equipment [PPE], etc.) in Hall A and C should be supported by power system, with installation of distribution box and electrical cabling nets. There should be a completely airtight space located in entrances in every semi-contaminated area in Hall A and C.

(4) Washrooms and bathrooms should be set up in Hall A, B and C. In Hall A, four washrooms are required for collecting filthy cloths, with 40 washing basins, and 40 portal electric water heaters. Moreover, two bathrooms are required with 12 sets of showering equipment and 40 portable electric water heaters. Whereas in Hall B and C, four washrooms are required with 40 washing basins and 40 portable electric water heaters. Moreover, two bathrooms are required, with 12 sets of showering equipment and 12 portable electric water heaters. Every room should be supported by lightning system, with

installation of cabling nets. Power should be provided for disinfection facilities and ventilation system. Distribution boxes and cabling nets should be provided for exterior sewage system.

(5) The exterior water supply system reconstruction: main water supply pipe should use DN100 PE which is connected with branch pipes of water container, matching valves, etc.

(6) The exterior drainage system reconstruction: main water drainage pipe should use DN150 UPVC. The entrance of parking basement in Hall A and C should be placed with 75m³ glass-made septic tank. The sewage systems are installed both in Hall A and C, which should be complemented with four sets of submersible sewage pumps, two control panels, and supporting valve equipment.

(7) Mechanical air supply and air exhaust systems should be installed in Hall A and C, with supporting distribution boxes and cabling nets.

(8) The ward areas in Hall A, B and C should be separated clearly by belts made in incombustible material and should be artistic and able to protect the privacy of patients.

3.2 Requirements for Reconstruction

3.2.1 Site Selection Requirements

The property chosen to reconstruct into Fangcang Shelter Hospitals should be single-floor or multi-floors. The standard of construction structure, fire resistance level, fire compartment, firefighting facilities and fire lanes should comply and follow the existing relevant regulations.

The location of Fangcang Shelter Hospitals should be away from urban, crowded zones such as CBD, schools or residential areas, as well as factories containing flammable and combustible materials and hazardous chemicals. Signs and indications should be placed in areas beside the Fangcang Shelter Hospital. A green belt should be placed between hospitals and surrounding buildings, to separate them by at least 20m. When actual conditions are not in favor in building the green belt, the distance between hospitals and surrounding buildings should be no less than 30m.

There should be a parking lot and turning spaces for ambulances, located at the entrance of the reconstructed property. The space should be sufficient for immediate evacuation, where ambulance can approach the outside traffic easily, but also directly connect to the internal control center. There should be extra rooms for medical support equipment, barrier free facilities, and logistics services in the parking lot. Moreover, the parking lot should also be provided with temporary tents and mobile medical facilities such as CT rooms and examination rooms, and basic facilities such as mobile toilets, washrooms and bathrooms. The interior space of the property should be easily separated into different zones using belts.

Public venues with good firefighting facilities, including exhibition centers, indoor stadiums, vacant factories, multi-function sports halls are preferred.

3.2.2 Reconstruction Structure

If the construction design of Fangcang Shelter Hospitals involves changing the original loadbearing of the buildings, a further evaluation and examination should be carried out by structural engineers. Precautions should be taken according to the actual situation and loadbearing adjustments made. Cautions should be taken in the following aspects:

(1) When transferring heavy weight medical equipment, evaluation on the layout plan and construction drawings should be carried out based on the loadbearing information. Precautions should be made according to actual condition, and site evaluation results (the weight of the equipment should be less than the loadbearing, increase the loadbearing accordingly).

(2) When setting up the separation belt between different areas, re-examination should be carried out based on the layout drawings and original loadbearing of the building. Precautions should be taken accordingly, for example using a lighter material for the separation belts.

(3) When transferring heavy mobile facilities and equipment, re-examinations should be carried out based on the actual weight of the equipment and its mobile path. Precautions should be taken accordingly.

(4) The separation belts should be installed safely and stably, and be tightly linked to each other.

3.2.3 Firefight Facilities Requirement

(1) All existing firefighting equipment should be accessible and should function normally. The lightning system for evacuation should be in a good condition. Indications should be placed on the floor for clarity in guiding the staff and patients to evacuate the building. Existing emergency exits should fulfill the relevant firefighting regulations and standards.

(2) Type A portable ammonium phosphate dry powder extinguisher should be equipped in the building. Severe hazardous area should be equipped at least with 3A level extinguisher, where the maximum area covered should be 50m². The powder used should be ammonium phosphate MF/ABC5. The extinguishers in the building should be secured and placed according to relevant regulations.

(3) Fire extinguishers should be equipped in valuable equipment storage room, treatment rooms and information system control rooms.

(4) If domestic water supply system is installed under the condition where there is no fire hose reel, there should be an extra hose reel equipped in the building (a portable fire hydrant is also applicable). The placement of such facilities should ensure the ratio of number of hydrant and surface area is 1:1.

(5) Every medical staff should be provided with a filtering respiratory protective equipment. Its placement should be clearly seen and easily accessed.

(6) A small-scale firefighting station should be set beside the nurse duty room, equipped with a portable high-pressure water mist with a capacity of 100ml.

(7) If condition allows, all fire alarm and firefighting linkage control system should be ensured to work reliably.

3.2.4 Requirements on the Construction Site

The designing process, purchasing process, construction and acceptance process should be carried out simultaneously. There should be a close working relationship established between the design team and construction team, which allows them to cooperate with each other and deliver an outstanding service and performance.

Different teams should be assigned to different zones and divisions, which take a modular approach, and deliver a standardized work performance. Duplicated work should be avoided, and reasonable time gaps should be provided in between different construction tasks.

Separation walls should be built based on the layout plans and construction drawings. Materials used for the walls should be light and incombustible, where the flammability should be low and no less than level B1. Acceptance check should be carried out area by area in a timely manner. Examinations and tests should be presented on the rigidity, strength, stability and leakproofness of the separation walls.

There should be extra precaution measures taken to increase the stability and strength of the walls, on supporting pipes and inside the separation walls. Walls and ceilings using light materials should be equipped with extra anti-cracking techniques.

Regular examination should be carried out on the ventilation system, power system and other related installed systems, to ensure that all systems installed fulfill the instructions on the designed plans and follow the guidance on relevant regulations and standards.

Precaution measures should be taken to ensure a healthy, clean working environment for staff on-site and extra care should be provided to decrease the risk of infection. There should be an infrared detector at every entrance and exit, supervised by staff who are responsible for manual testing on staffs' body temperature. Randomized check on staffs' body temperature should be done every four hours.

The toilets and offices for staffs should be disinfected every six hours. Keep the working sites clean and maintain the room ventilation in a good condition.

Smoking is strictly prohibited in working sites. Extra precaution should be made to emphasize firefighting management. Decrease the use of open flame in the working site if it is possible. Install extinguishers and small-scale firefighting station in the building according to the regulations.

A spare dual power system should be installed in the building. Every area should be equipped with an electric leakage protection device, to ensure the safety of the working and site and construction.

3.3 Reconstruction of Water Supply and Drainage

3.3.1 Construction Design Principle

Constructions should be carried out based on the construction drawings and other relevant information drawings provided by the construction company. Reconstruction should strictly comply and follow the relevant regulations and standards.

3.3.2 Water Supply System

Water supply system in the Fangcang Shelter Hospitals should be reconstructed in the base of existing water supplying pipe in the property. An extra pressure-reducing and anti-backflow device should be installed in the entrance of water pipe in order to prevent the polluted water flow backward. Alternatively, a break tank could be used for water supplying. Water pressure should be maintained in at least 0.25Mpa. Extra ports for domestic water pressure and chlorination should be reserved. Flushing and disinfection devices should be equipped in the parking lots for ambulances. For interior water supply pipes, S3.2, PPR should be used with hot-melt conjunction. For interior hot water supply pipe, S2.5, PPT should be used with hot-melt conjunction. For water pipe with DN<50mm of diameter, copper stop valve should be used; for DN>50mm, high-temperature resistance stop valve should be installed on hot water supply pipes. The copper-core valve with ductile cast iron shell should be installed on pressure drainage pipe, with a nominal pressure of 100MPa.

3.3.3 Water Heating System

Electric water heating system should be implemented in the bathrooms, with devices to ensure ground protection, so as to prevent burning, high pressure and overheating. Extra precaution measures should be taken to prevent situation including electric leakage, and automatic power cuts.

3.3.4 Water Boiling System

Each ward area should be complemented with a boiling water supply station, for provision of adequate drinking water and boiling water, in a timely manner. The drinking water quality should adhere to the local "Sanitary Standard for Drinking Water". Alternatively, if water boiling system is not feasible, it can be replaced with water dispenser.

3.3.5 Drainage System

Proper disinfection must be applied on disposed feces, vomitus, sewage and medical liquid waste. Solid medical waste and chemicals cannot be directly disposed into sewer before disinfection. It is strictly prohibited to dispose medical wastes and sewage from polluted areas into the sewer, without being disinfected.

Proper disinfection must be applied on domestic sewage from temporary toilets. Sewage must be collected centrally, and the disinfection procedure must comply with relevant domestic disposal regulations and standards. The water quality of disinfected sewage has to meet the "Standards of Disposed Water Pollutants of Medical Institutions" based on the local standards. The disinfection procedure is shown as below:

(1) After the use of temporary toilets, immediately put an appropriate number of disinfectant tablets (peracetic acid, sodium hypochlorite or bleaching powder) into the toilets. The sewage should be collected centrally by local environment department, which are then transported to sewage disposal station and disinfected. It is prohibited to directly dispose the polluted sewage into urban drainage pipe network.

(2) The sewage from ward areas should be collected centrally, which will then be disposed into the nearby septic tank. The liquid medical waste shall be distributed into existing drainage inspection tanks. Liquid medical waste and sewage from ward areas should be disposed through separate drainage pipes, into separate septic tanks.

(3) Sewage from Fangcang Shelter Hospitals should undergo disinfection procedure twice before being distributed into urban drainage pipes. For properties equipped with three-compartment

septic tanks: put appropriate amount of disinfection tablets into one of the compartments, which will then be distributed outwards after at least 15 hours; disinfect the sewage for the second time at the entrance of the urban drainage pipe. The condition of the sewage should meet the requirement and standards set by local environment department.

(4) The duration of the exposure of sewage to liquid chloride, chlorine dioxide, sodium hypochlorite, bleaching powder or calcium hypochlorite should be at least 15 hours, with residual chlorine more than 6.5mg/L, fecal coliform smaller than 100/L and choline dosage of 50mg/L. If the required duration of exposure is not feasible, the dosage of residual chlorine and available chlorine should be increased.

(5) For properties without any sewage disposal or treatment facilities, temporary sewage collection tank or mobile septic tank should be installed, which allow the hospital to efficiently dispose any polluted liquid.

(6) Ventilation pipes installed above the ceiling should be equipped with high-efficiency filter or UV disinfection device. The equipment should be provided by mobile toilet suppliers.

(7) Sewage from vehicle wash station and disinfected wastewater should be disposed though drainage pipe. Sewage effluent should

be sealed with proper facilities. Moveable mechanical piston is prohibited in sealing the effluent. The water depth should not be less than 50mm.

3.3.6 Installation of Drainage System

For Fangcang Shelter Hospitals drainage pipes, UPVs should be used, with plastic cement. Bathrooms should be equipped with straight floor or grid-type floor drain. Water storage space should be reserved below the drain, with depth of no less than 50mm. When connecting sanitary facilities, which has no water storage space, with domestic drainage pipe or other pipes which may produce poisoned gas, there should be water storage space below the sewage effluent. The depth for water storage should not be less than 50mm. Drainage pipes should be installed following the instructions below, otherwise comply with the specifications shown in construction drawings.

**Standard slopes for installation of drainage pipes
of Fangcang Shelter Hospital**

Pipe size	DN75	DN100	DN150	DN200
Standard slopes for installation of sewage and waste water pipes	0.025	0.020	0.02	0.01

45° tee, 45° cross, 90° lateral tee or 90° lateral cross must be used between horizontal pipes and between horizontal pipes and vertical pipes of drainage pipelines.

3.3.7 Sanitary Facilities

Automatic or touchless faucet sinks should be installed in every water-use site and sanitary facilities with sterility standards, or facilities which are used for epidemic prevention and control. Measures should be taken in order to prevent the splashing of water or dirt. The following water-use sites should be equipped with automatic or touchless faucet sinks:

(1) Basins for medical staff: including sinks and test tanks in bacteriological laboratory.

(2) Public toilets: Urinal and pedestal pan should be provided with automatic sensor faucets, while squatting pots should be provided with foot-pedal faucets or automatic sensor faucets.

(3) Basins for hand washing: Touchless faucets or foot-pedal faucets should be used.

3.4 Reconstruction of Ventilation and Air Conditioning

3.4.1 The Importance and Necessity of Ventilation System Installation

The existing ventilation and air condition systems installed in the properties before reconstruction into Fangcang Shelter Hospitals are mostly positive pressure systems, which will fail to meet a medical institution's requirements and standards. The principle of reconstruction of ventilation and air condition system is to design and install additional facilities and devices to existing systems, to change the working mechanisms of the systems, which allows different areas to have different room pressures. Always ensure the highest room pressure in clean areas, and lowest room pressure in contaminated areas.

3.4.2 Construction Model

In order to accelerate the rate of reconstruction process, and to fulfill the design requirements, the integrative reconstruction approach "engineer-procure-construct" (also known as EPC) can be adopted. While the engineering and construction contractor carry out the detailed engineering design of the project and procure all the equipment and materials necessary, they should also construct to deliver a functioning facility or asset into the existing property. There should be a close working relationship and efficient communication established between the design team, purchase team and construction team in the designing stage: site investigations should be carried out, meanwhile all the functional facilities and materials should be prepared, with a detailed working schedule formulate by the construction team. When entering the construction stage, designers should carry out in-site services, in order to adjust designing plans according to actual conditions.

3.4.3 Ventilation System Design Key Points

(1) Mechanical air supply and air exhaust systems should be installed in contaminated and semi-contaminated areas. Air should go through a high efficiency filter before exhausting. The filter should be placed in the entrance of exhaust blowers. Mechanical air supply and air exhaust systems can be installed in clean areas, alternatively, open air spaces for natural ventilation.

(2) Central air conditioning system for contaminated and semi-contaminated area should be equipped with air cleaning and disinfection devices. When it is feasible, higher-efficiency filter can be installed in the air conditioning machine. UV disinfection lamps can be installed near the return air filter and surface air coolers.

(3) Temporary air ventilation and exhaust facilities should be installed in the existing property based on construction drawings.

The air flow direction should be from medical staff working areas to ward areas. There should be no dead corners left where air cannot be circulated properly.

(4) When existing air conditioning and ventilation systems is usable, they should be reset to DC air supply and exhaust system. Return air valves should be turned off, while air damper should be opened in full set. Full fresh air should be circulated into interior space, with the rate of exhausting larger than rate of supplying. If existing air conditioning and ventilation system is not feasible, or there is no ventilation system installed in the existing property, there should be additional functional facilities equipped during the reconstruction. Cabinet fans with appropriate air volume and a suitable wind pressure should be installed to complement the existing systems. The height of the cabinet should be no taller than 2m, while equipped with precaution controlling measure. The air conditioning and ventilation system should work 24/7.

(5) The exhaust air rate should be set to 150m³/h per person.

(6) When medical staff passing through clean areas and contaminated areas: the air supply rate in the first changing room should be no less than 30 times/h. D300 ventilation pipes should be used in between the changing rooms and buffer rooms. When the medical staff return from contaminated zone to clean zone, the air exhaust rate in the buffer room and room for removing PPE should not be less than 30

times per hour. D300 ventilation pipe should be used in between changing rooms and buffer rooms. The direction of air flow should be from clean zones to contaminated zones.

(7) There should be functional facilities of sterilization and disinfection equipped in every isolated ward area. Additional heating system should also be installed based on actual conditions.

(8) Emergency temporary dry toilets should be provided in isolated ward areas. Additional air exhaustion system should be installed in toilets for medical staff. The exhaustion rate should not be less than 12 times/h. High-efficiency filter should be equipped at the entrance of exhaustion outlets.

(9) The construction of ventilation and exhaustion system should be adjusted according to the actual situation; always ensure that fresh air circulates from outside. The outside environment near fresh air supply outlet should be clean and free from contamination. Outdoor exhaustion outlet should be installed in high altitude. The position should be above any supplying outlets by a minimum of 20m, while the horizontal separation distance between exhaustion and supplying outlet should not be less than 6m.

3.5 Reconstruction of Electrical and Intelligence System

(1) Ventilation system should be centralized controlled in nursing

station (on-call room). Relevant equipment should be supplied in a full set.

(2) Light intensity should be adjusted in the reconstructed property to reduce glare impacts. Additional lamps can be installed on the walls of the open spaces, alternatively, upright light can be installed on the floor. Non-transparent covers should be provided on the lamps or using indirect illumination facilities.

(3) There should be sufficient wireless network coverage, ensuring the accessibility of 4G and 5G network. When it is feasible, there should be provision of AP and WIFI network.

(4) Additional lamps, electricity wires and LV lines should be covered in metallic conduits or metal trunkings. The position of such conduits and trunkings should be set away from corridors. Precaution measures should be taken in order to prevent any incontinence caused by them.

(5) Sockets for UV sterilizer and air freshener should be installed in bathroom and buffer rooms. Power should be supplied through reserved electric circuits. The sockets for UV sterilizers should be indicated clearly and be separated from those for lightning.

(6) Medical equipment rooms, bathrooms, and any functional rooms where people can bath, should be equipped with supplementary

equipotential bonding facilities.

(7) Alarm bottom should be positioned in nursing station (duty room). The signal should be directed to security staff station.

(8) CCTV should be installed in medical staff areas and ward areas.

(9) Projector and screen should be provided in each resting and entertainment area, for social engagement needs.

(10) When it is feasible, power sockets should be installed on the separation belt beside the ward beds. Insulation inspections should be carried out at least once before conducting electricity through wires. The insulation resistance testing voltage and insulation resistance between LV/ELV power circuit and lines in the grounds, should be no less than 0.5Ω.

3.6 Ward Settings

There should be negative pressure in the ward area which is set by the ventilation system. The exhaustion rate should be set at no less than $200m^3/hxp$. Air should go through a low-efficiency filter (G4), followed by medium-efficiency filter (F8) and a high-efficiency filter (H11) before exhausting though a vertical pipe positioned at height. The external door (the doors in the wards are mostly double-layered) should be frequently opened, in order to supplement air, using negative pressure.

The suppliers should deliver the ventilation and exhaustion pipes which are equipped with fabric air ducts. The outdoor exhaustion outlet should be positioned no lower than eave. A rodent-resistant net should be installed in the entrance of the exhaustion outlet. The gap between each ventilation machine and doors, should be sealed properly.

Electrical air cleanser and fresher should be placed in the main corridors in ward areas and medical staff working areas.

3.6.1 Buffer Room Settings

Ventilation and exhaustion systems should be installed in buffer rooms. The air supply rate in the first changing room should be 30 times/h. A gate should be placed in between the first changing room and second changing room, in order to convey air from first changing room to second changing room. Ventilation and exhaustion system should be installed in bathrooms and PPE doffing rooms.

High-efficiency filters and should be installed in the ventilation system. The size of the pipe should be D110, which is integrated by metal bellows and UPVC pipes.

3.6.2 Other Configurations

Temporary bathrooms and shower places placed outside the Fangcang Shelter Hospitals should be provided with ventilation and exhaustion systems, which is equipped with high-efficiency filter. The size of the pipe should be D110, which is integrated by metal bellows and UPVC pipes. The exhaustion rate should be set at 8 times/h.

3.7 The Setting-up of Hardware and Software

3.7.1 Hardware Settings

Interior settings: The hardware requirements inside the Fangcang Shelter Hospitals would be mainly ward beds. It is highly suggested to use dorm-use or army-use bunk beds or foldable beds. Disinfection procedures can be applied, which can be also separated by physical belts made from eco-friendly materials. It is also necessary to have sufficient number of quilts, mats and other bedding staff. If interior temperature is low, electrical blankets and hot pads should also be provided to medical staffs and patients. If it is feasible, 5G network should cover the hospitals, to provide convenience in telecommunication.

Exterior settings: High-end medical technology equipment should be provided, which include vans for imaging examinations, testings, rescue works and P3 laboratory works.

3.7.2 Human Resource Management and Software Settings

The ratio between patient number and number of medical staff, cleaning staff and food delivery staff should be reasonable and sufficient. Taking Zall (Wuhan Salon) Fangcang Shelter Hospital as an example, in total there are 1169 medical staff, made up by 22 medical professional teams, accompanied by 15 nurse teams and 1 radiologic technologist team nationwide. Hierarchical management adopted in managing the medical staff divides medical staffs into four levels: director of medical affairs, director of hall, director of shelter, and doctors. There are, in total, four shifts that changes every six hours per day, namely A, P, N1 and N2. Each medical staff will have one day-off after working for two days. Every shift should be made up by one doctor and five nurses, who are responsible for taking care of approximately 100 patients.

Apart from medical staffs, there should also be staffs responsible for food delivery, security, cleaning, disinfection, psychological intervention, and heat and electricity maintenance. Take Zall (Wuhan Salon) Fangcang Shelter Hospital as an example: there are in total approximately 100 people in logistic support team. Within the team, there are 54 cleaning staff (three shifts) who are responsible for disposing domestic and medical wastes which weighted 600-700kg per day.

Chapter 4

Fangcang Shelter Hospitals Operation Model

4.1 General Rules and Principles

4.1.1 Management Principles

Management principles include: targeted admission, centralized isolation, division management by units, standardized treatment procedure, and "two-way" referral.

4.1.2 Operation Objectives

To avoid cross infection, treat mild COVID-19 patients from community in an isolated environment while controlling sources of infection. In the meantime, provide various education program on COVID-19, as well as psychological consulting session, in order to maintain the mental stability of the patients. Frequent monitoring and treatment should be provided to patients in a timely manner to prevent the patients' conditions from getting worse and decreasing mortality.

4.1.3 Organizational Structure

The Fangcang Shelter Hospitals are controlled and organized under a unified epidemic prevention and control center. The president of the hospital is fully responsible for its operation and management, and the vice-president is responsible for coordination and cooperation. Staff are divided into different teams and assigned with specific jobs and tasks:

(1) Integrated Information and Data Control Team (with assigned team leader): Preparation of operation schemes: determination of workflow; overall human resources management on division of labor and coordination; collecting, analysing and reporting of various useful information; cooperation and coordination on transferring; scheduling of administration and induction of medical and logistic staff; and last but not least, coordination on operation issues.

(2) Medical Operation Team (with assigned team leader): Consists of medical groups and nursing groups. The medical groups are responsible for preparing healthcare plans, developing relevant core systems and processes, summarizing the information of medical staff profile and scheduling for them. The nursing groups are responsible for arranging nursing workflow and SOPs, including preparing nursing plans and processes, summarizing the information of nurses' profiles, and scheduling for them.

(3) Epidemic Prevention and Control Team (with assigned team leader): Responsible for preparation and implementation of a prevention and control system, provision of relevant training programs, and nosocomial infection surveillance and monitoring during operation.

(4) Logistics Support Team (with assigned team leader): Responsible for efficiently allocating the medical and living resources and supplies, including providing medical equipment and facilities, preparation of medicines, environmental sanitation, disposal of medical waste, sewage discharge etc.

(5) Moreover, a functional management board can be established for each hospital. The size and function can be determined based on the actual situation and circumstances.

4.1.4 Working Mechanism

Each team should have a clear division of function, which should be suitable for its own workflow and responsibility. Assign members into different shifts and plan the schedule according to the assigned shifts, then implement the system comprehensively. Besides, each team leader shall be responsible for the internal and external communication, coordination, information reporting and emergency situations to address the various problems that arise from the operations.

A scheduling system based on different time periods, shift change management system, and summary and report systems should be implemented.

4.1.5 Work Discipline

(1) Be subject to overall command, have clear division of function, act proactively, and support each other.

(2) Ensure unobstructed communication and keep the phones available 24/7.

(3) Be punctual. Otherwise, please report in advance if there is a reasonable excuse to do so.

(4) Do not disclose any confidential information in any inappropriate circumstance.

4.2 Admission Criteria

Taking account of the actual situation, the health condition of patients being admitted in Fangcang Shelter Hospitals should meet the following criteria:

(1) Present mild symptoms (mild clinical signs and symptoms, no evidence of pneumonia on imaging tests) or common symptoms (fever, respiratory symptoms or other symptoms, evidence of pneumonia on imaging tests).

(2) No clear functional disability.

(3) No evidence of severe chronic diseases (CHD), malignant tumors, structural lung diseases, pulmonary heart diseases and immunosuppression.

(4) No history of mental illness.

(5) Do not have blood oxygen saturation (SpO_2) > 93% over a blood testing on finger, and a respiratory rate <30bpm when resting.

(6) Any other medical history and condition(s) should be clearly specified and explained.

4.3 Admission Procedure and Policy

(1) Before 10 a.m. every day, the head of the nursing group (head nurse) in each admission area of patients reports the number of patients that can be transferred to the director of the hospital office, according to the status of available beds. Then the director of the hospital office contacts the vice-president to determine the number of patients to be received on the same day and reports to the Epidemic Prevention and Control Command Center.

(2) According to the available ward bed capacity and admission capacity provided by the Epidemic Prevention and Control Center,

it should then confirm and provide the information of the number of patients, along with their profiles, to Fangcang Shelter Hospitals.

(3) Each Fangcang Shelter Hospital should establish a panel to review the status of the patients according to the admission standards, which helps in determining the list of patients to be received, as well as the bed number assigned to them. A proof certificate should be issued for the transfer of every patient, and the Control Center should be informed of the transfers.

(4) Epidemic Prevention and Control Center is responsible for printing the information profile of each patients along with their Patient ID, which should be delivered to the patients alongside with the Transfer Certificate.

(5) Epidemic Prevention and Control Center should arrange for the transfer of patients, coordinate ambulance dispatch and entourages on board, as well as manage the information of the ambulances. The patients' ID and their Transfer Certificate should be placed on the ambulance.

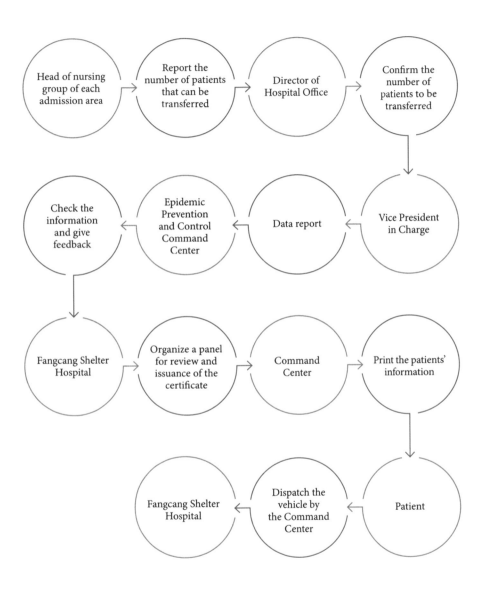

Fig. 4-1 Admission Procedure Chart of Fangcang Shelter Hospital

4.4 Pre-Examination and Triage

Fangcang Shelter Hospitals arrange medical staffs to carry out pre-examination and triage for patients. After pre-examination and relevant medical tests, the medical staff should give guidance to the patients who meet the admission criteria for hospitalization in a timely manner. The principle of "admission first, referral later" should be followed when handling patients who do not meet the admission criteria while still presenting severe symptoms. To ensure medical safety, patients considered as severe cases should first be placed in the observation areas, then provided with timely treatment as well as frequent monitoring on their health conditions. Medical staff should contact designated hospitals and arrange the referral immediately.

4.5 Daily Health Check on Patients

Closely monitor the vital signs and oxygen saturation as per the following procedure:

(1) Measure and record body temperature four times a day at 8 a.m., 12 a.m., 4 p.m. and 8 p.m.

(2) Record respiratory rate (RR) twice a day, at 8 a.m. and 8 p.m.

(3) Measure heart rate (HR) and finger blood oxygen saturation twice a day at 8a.m. and 8p.m.; patients who have shown an unstable

result may be applied with a finger clip oximeter to detect the transcutaneous oxygen saturation; frequent monitoring on oxygen saturation is required for patients with the severe disease until the conditions are relieved. Alternatively, patients should be transferred to a designated hospital.

(4) Whether to conduct laboratory tests or imaging tests is decided by the responsible physician according to the patient's condition.

(5) Whether to perform special examinations is decided by the responsible physician according to the patient's condition.

4.6 Intensive Care on Severe Patients

Severe patients refer to those who have been seriously ill at admission and mild patients whose conditions exacerbated during hospitalization period. In each ward area, there should be additional space for severe patents, which allows medical staff to closely monitor on them and provide timely treatment. The space shall be equipped with oxygen cylinders, rescue ambulance, rescue medicine, simple respirators, and monitoring and rescue equipment, as well as non-invasive ventilator and transfer wagon (where possible). A specially assigned medical staff should be responsible for the area and allocation of the medical staff should be strengthened and prioritized.

4.6.1 Indications for Consultation and Transferring to the Observation Area of Severe Patients

(1) Continuous subjective symptoms without alleviation, or patients' conditions continuously worsen.

(2) Consistent water intake and physical cooling measures when body temperature is under 38°C. If the temperature keeps rising, then consultation and transfer should be initiated.

(3) RR ≥ 30 bpm, oxygen inhalation, not relieved;

(4) Finger blood oxygen saturation ≤ 93%;

(5) HR ≥ 100bpm, BP ≥ 140/90mmHg; patients with hypertension are treated by taking antihypertensive drugs orally on a regular basis; patients with hypertension do not get improved after oxygen inhalation and antipyretic treatment.

4.6.2 Rescue Procedure for Severe Patients

(1) Transfer the patients to the observation and treatment area of severe cases using wheelchairs or wagons;

(2) Evaluate the state of illness, open the intravenous channels and implement treatment;

(3) Provide life support and conduct monitoring;

(4) Apply to transfer the patients to the designated hospitals by reporting to the Command Center according to the above transfer procedures;

(5) Record the actual situation and report.

4.6.3 Transfer Standards for Severe Patients

In principle, patients who show one of the following symptoms are considered for transfer:

(1) Respiratory distress, RR>30bpm;

(2) Oxygen saturation <93% at rest;

(3) Arterial partial pressure of oxygen (PaO_2) / fraction of inspired oxygen (FiO_2) <300mmHg (1mmHg = 0.133kPa);

(4) The lesion shows a significant progression of >50% within 24 to 48 hours as shown in a lung imaging;

(5) Patients with combined severe chronic diseases, including hypertension, diabetes, coronary heart diseases, malignant tumor, structural lung diseases, pulmonary heart disease and immunosuppression.

(6) Other reasonable specific reasons.

4.6.4 Transfer Procedure for Severe Patients

Patients in Fangcang Shelter Hospitals with unstable health conditions, or who meet the transferring criteria mentioned in previous section, should first be consulted by doctors in the specific area. After consultation, they can be transferred following the procedure below:

(1) The senior doctors will provide consultation to the patients after relevant examination and triage, together with the responsible physician who accompany the patients from the start.

(2) Patients who are confirmed as severe case after consultation, shall be reported to the Command Center immediately and transferred to the designated hospitals for more comprehensive treatment;

(3) Complete the transfer register form and wait for further induction from Command Center;

(4) Coordinate to complete the handover process based on the instruction given; arrange medical staff to escort the transfer wagon, as well as keep the medical record of the patients updated.

4.7 Discharge Criteria and Procedure

4.7.1 Discharge Criteria

Patients can be discharged once the health conditions have met the following indications:

(1) Body temperature is stable over three days;

(2) Significant improvement of respiratory symptoms;

(3) Clear absorption of inflammation as shown in lung imaging;

(4) Positive results of two consecutive (with at least 24 hours interval) NAT of respiratory pathogen;

Patients showing the above indications can be discharged from the Fangcang Shelter Hospital after getting consent from both specialist and head doctor after mutual agreement from consultation.

4.7.2 Discharge Procedure

(1) The senior doctors will provide consultation to the patients after relevant examination and consultation issued by responsible physician.

(2) Patients who meet the discharge criteria should be reported to the Command Center in a timely manner.

(3) Complete the discharge form and wait for the further instructions, coordinate to complete the handover process based on the instructions given.

(4) Arrange medical staff to escort the discharged, as well as keep the medical records of the patients updated.

(5) A clear explanation must be given to the discharged patients on the necessary home-quarantine: self-isolation in a single room while wearing a mask. Going out is forbidden. Body temperature must be measured every day during the 14-day home quarantine. For patients who fall under the condition where home-quarantine is not feasible, they should follow the instructions and centralized quarantine arranged by Command Center. If the patients start to show COVID-19 symptoms again, or experience worsening of conditions, their conditions should be reported to the person-in-charge of the community immediately. The patients should immediately seek for medical intervention in a designated hospital.

4.8 Disinfection and Disposal Procedure

On the day of discharge, patients may bring along their personal belongings; at the exit of the ward area, patients shall disinfect their upper outer garments and pants by spraying 75% ethyl alcohol, step on a foot mat containing chlorine disinfectant (2000 mg/l) and wash their hands with disinfectant.

For patients who meet the requirements for bathing (evaluation required), the clothes they have worn and the supplies they have used should be disinfected by spraying 75% ethyl alcohol. It is recommended that the clothes and supplies be disposed of as medical waste and handed over to the cleaning staff for centralized incineration; For patients who are unwilling to destroy their clothes, suppliers can pack the items in double-layer garbage bags after disinfection and let them take home for disposal.

Prepare one clean mask for each discharged patient who shall wear the mask from the contaminated area into the clean area; at the exit of the clean area, patients shall again disinfect their upper outer garments and pants by spraying 75% ethyl alcohol, step on a foot mat containing chlorine disinfectant (2000 mg/l) and wash their hands with disinfectant.

Destroy the sheets, beddings, and other items that have been used by the patients after disinfection. Disinfect the surface of the mattresses, bedside tables, chairs, and thermos that have been used by the patients, so that the articles can be used by the newly admitted patients. Provide new beddings and sheets for newly admitted patients.

Fig. 4-2 Disinfection Process for Discharged Patients of Fangcang Shelter Hospital

Chapter 5

Fangcang Shelter Hospitals Logistics Support

To provide logistics support for Fangcang shelter hospitals, we formulate the following plans from the aspects of catering, accommodation, cleaning, and supplies, based on actual logistic situations.

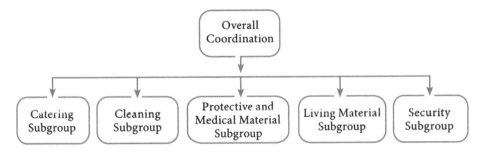

Fig. 5-1 Logistics Support Chart of Fangcang Shelter Hospital

5.1 Materials and Supplies Support

5.1.1 Catering Support

5.1.1.1 Staffing

One manager in charge of providing contact information and coordinating with other departments.

5.1.1.2 Work plan

(1) Count the number of patients and staff on a daily basis, prepare meals in advance, and ensure that they are sufficient.

(2) Distribute food according to the name list and preplanned timeline.

(3) Contact catering company.

(4) Ensure cleanliness, safety and hygiene.

(5) Ensure daily delivery of fresh food and food safety. Impose strict quantity and quality check.

(6) Suggested breakfast time is 7:00 to 8:00, lunch time is 11:30 to 12:30, and dinner time is 17:30 to 18:30.

5.1.1.3 Requirement

(1) Send the catered food for patients and medical workers to the designated area, and notify them in a communication group, by broadcast, or through other means of communication.

(2) Summarize the distribution of breakfast, lunch and dinner to patient and staff.

5.1.2 Hygiene Support

5.1.2.1 Staffing

Two managers in charge of providing contact information and coordinating with other departments.

5.1.2.2 Work plan

(1) Arrange cleaning worker of each area, including public areas, patient areas, clean areas, toilets/ washrooms and other locations.

(2) Assign cleaners based on demand. Dispose of garbage in time.

(3) Redeploy and reallocate staff when needed.

(4) Guide patients to ensure their personal hygiene.

5.1.2.3 Requirement

(1) Clean up after breakfast, lunch, and dinner on a regular basis. Enforce rectification if the requirement is not met. Require the cleaning staff to sign in at the responsible area every hour.

(2) Garbage cleaning. Provide access to garbage bins such as on walkways, doorways, dining areas or each floor. And the cleaning staff should move the garbage to the garbage room in a timely manner.

5.1.3 Medical Supplies Support

5.1.3.1 Staffing

Two managers in charge of providing contact information and coordinating with other departments.

5.1.3.2 Work plan

(1) Make lists and ensure the supplies of personal protective equipment according to the daily schedule of doctors and nurses.

(2) Register the usage of protective equipment according to the temporary work arrangement. All PPE should be received within hours to avoid wasting.

(3) Keep records of the collection of protective clothing and ensure the record is accurate and consistent.

(4) Set up special protective materials distribution posts with 24 hours shift. Supplies such as oxygen bottles and medicines shall be provided to the patient whenever necessary.

5.1.3.3 Requirements

(1) When the inventory of protective materials is less than 100 sets (the specific standard depends on the number of medical personnel in the shelter), report and coordinate immediately.

(2) At the distribution office, explain the correct use of protective materials and avoid cross infection.

(3) At the distribution office, the recipient should report their name and sign before receiving the materials, according to the shift and the schedule.

5.1.4 Life Supply Support

5.1.4.1 Staffing

Two managers in charge of providing contact information and coordinating with other departments.

5.1.4.2 Work plan

(1) Provide patients with sufficient daily necessities such as quilts, electric blankets, cups, pots, towels, etc.

(2) Coordinate the supply of water, electricity, network, etc. to ensure that patients have hot water and electric power available.

(3) Arrange the working area, including office supplies such as computers, stationery, tables and chairs.

(4) Connect with the donation office to ensure that the donated materials are stored and distributed safely, and make the best use of the donated items.

5.1.4.3 Requirement

(1) The registration list shall be completed according to the bed number of the patient when the supply is collected.

(2) Count the distribution of materials to ensure that the items are sufficient.

5.1.5 Management of Medicine

5.1.5.1 Formulate a drug catalog for Fangcang Shelter Hospital

According to the characteristics of the patients admitted in the hospital, combined with the relevant diagnosis and treatment plans and guidelines, and comprehensive clinical front-line expert opinions, evaluate and analyze the drug needs for the hospital's COVID-19 treatment. The catalog should be mainly composed of drugs for symptomatic treatment, prevention of complications, basic diseases and first aid. The final list of drugs is determined by the clinical pharmacist and purchasing department. In the later stage, according to the actual clinical situation, regularly adjust the quantity and variety of drugs.

The catalog includes the following medicine:

(1) Antiviral, antibacterial, analgesic-antipyretic, antitussive, antiasthmatic and expectorant, gastrointestinal drugs;

(2) Hypnotics and sedatives;

(3) Drugs for blood pressure or glucose reduction, lipid regulation and other chronic diseases;

(4) Chinese patent medicines or other traditional medicines clinically tested to be effective in the rehabilitation of COVID-19 patients;

(5) Drugs for first aid

5.1.5.2 Establishment of hospital pharmacy

Take Zall (Jianghan Wuzhan) Square Cabin Hospital as an example, the hospital pharmacy covers an area of about 30m² and is set in a clean zone and divided into qualified area, unqualified area and secondary storage area. The hospital is equipped with basic facilities such as computers, printers, fire protection, and anti-theft to ensure that the storage conditions of medicines meet the requirements of relevant management regulations.

5.1.5.3 Procurement and supply

Drug supply team is in charge of drugs, who should formulate unified procurement and request plans. The pharmaceutical emergency leading team determines the list of medicines to be procured urgently in accordance with the established hospital pharmacy drug catalog.

Other than ensuring common medical supplies, the hospital should also focus on ensuring adequate supply of drugs related to COVID-19 treatment and store the drug in specific areas. The purchase must be made from pharmaceutical companies with legal qualifications. The qualifications of relevant companies and business personnel must be recorded alongside the purchase for transparency and accountability. When there are shortage of supplies, the hospital should actively negotiate and communicate with the providers, encourage them to expand the supply chain or transfer the supplies from other regions. Meanwhile, if the purchasing process is difficult, the hospital should actively seek alternative supplies and materials and publish drug guidelines to the clinic.

5.1.5.4 Management of donated drugs

(1) Acceptance criteria for donated drugs:

1. For those produced within China, the drug must be a product approved by the local drug regulatory authority with a valid approval number, and meet quality standards. The drug must be valid and effective for at least 6 months.

2. For drugs produced outside China, the varieties should be approved and registered by local regulatory authorities, included in the international general pharmacopoeia, legally produced and marketed in registered countries, and meet quality standards; the expiry date is more than 6 months.

(2) Standard process for accepting donated medicines:

1. Formulate a list of donated medicines: Discuss and develop a list of medicines acceptable for donation and update them regularly. The medicines already in the catalogue can be accepted as donations directly.

2. Receiving process of donated drugs outside the catalog: After receiving the donated medicine, the drug supply group submits the product information and instructions provided by the donor to a clinical pharmacy for clinical demonstration and evaluation or consults the clinical medical team and clinical experts to determine whether to accept the donation.

3. Quantity of medicines accepted for donation: The amount of donated drug is determined by pharmaceutical emergency leadership team based on the usage of drugs, the time and the stage of the epidemic.

5.2 Living and Social Engagement Support

The shelter hospital servers as a "special community" for patients with mild disease. In order to enrich the cultural life of patients and enhance their courage to overcome the virus, it is recommended to set up in shelter hospital following the suggestion below:

(1) Reading corner: Each hospital is equipped with a bookshelf, where excellent books are placed for patients to read freely. See Fig. 5-2.

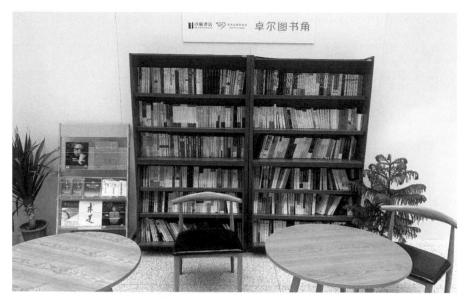

Fig. 5-2 Book Corner of Zall (North Hankou) Fangcang Shelter Hospital

(2) Food corner: Each hospital can set up a food corner with foods such as instant noodles, milk and fruits. See Fig. 5-3.

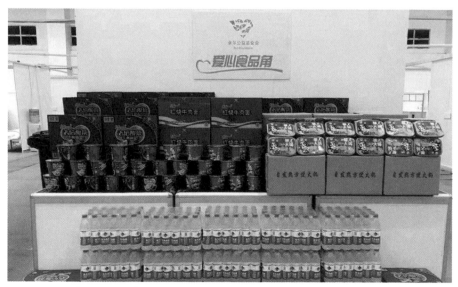

Fig. 5-3 Food Corner of Zall (Wuhan Salon) Fangcang Shelter Hospital

(3) Charging station: Each hospital should have one or more free charging stations for patients. See Fig. 5-4.

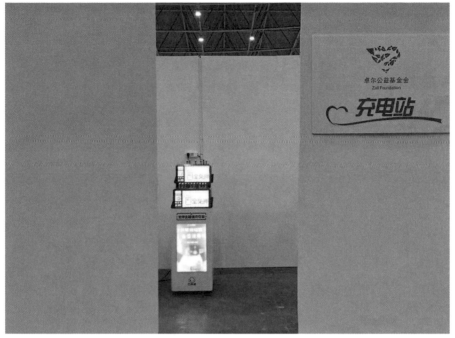

Fig. 5-4 Charging Station of Zall (Wuhan Salon) Fangcang Shelter Hospital

(4) Entertainment corner: For each hospital, install 1 or 2 televisions in the open space. On one hand, the corner can serve as an area for patients to watch various TV programs, on the other hand, the area can be used to organize square dance, game programs, poetry recitation, chorus and other literary programs to enrich patients' lives, and enhance their confidence and courage to overcome the virus. See Fig. 5-5 and Fig. 5-6.

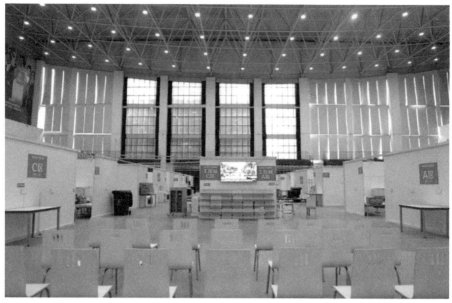

Fig. 5-5 Entertainment Corner of Zall (Wuhan Salon) Fangcang Shelter Hospital

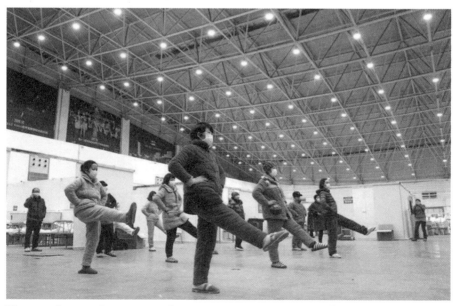

Fig. 5-6 Square Dancing at the Entertainment Corner of Zall (Wuhan Salon) Fangcang Shelter Hospital

(5) Psychological counseling: COVID-19 is a brand-new infectious disease. Its sudden attack brings a series of emergency disorders and anxieties to the patients. Thus, a certain amount of mental health counseling is required.

5.3 Safety Support

5.3.1 Medical Waste Management System for Fangcang Shelter Hospital

(1) Induction should be provided to manager at each level on the main responsibility. Attach great importance to the management of medical waste generated, and effectively implement the main responsibility. The person in charge of each district is the first person to be held responsible for medical waste management, and the operators who produced medical waste are the direct persons held responsible for the waste. Strengthen the effort for environmental sanitation and hygiene, dispose medical waste timely to avoid its accumulation, and strive to create a healthy and hygienic environment.

(2) Training system. All staff including physicians, nurses, technicians, administrators, and workers receive unified training from the Infection Control Team.

(3) Supervision system. The Infection Control Team is responsible for regular inspections and problems collection, feedbacks and

rectification supervision of the collection and treatment of medical waste in each zone.

(4) Be aware about the scope of items for collection. Waste produced by medical institutions or hospitals during the treatment of suspected or confirmed COVID-19 patients, including medical waste and garbage, should be collected, classified and disposed in the same way as medical waste.

(5) Establish strict standards for packaging and containers. Warning signs must be attached to the surface of special packaging bags and sharps containers for medical waste. Before disposing medical waste, careful inspection should be carried out to ensure the container is not damaged or leaking. Containers which are foot-operated and with lids are preferred for waste collection. When the medical waste reaches 3/4 of the packaging bag or sharps container, it should be sealed effectively and tightly. Double-layer packaging bags should be used to contain medical waste, and gooseneck-type seals should be used for layered sealing.

(6) Collect wastes safely. According to the type of medical waste, collect the waste in a timely manner, while ensuring the safety of personnel and minimising the risk of infection. When the surface of the packaging bag and sharps container is contaminated with infectious waste, a layer of packaging bag should be added. It is strictly forbidden to squeeze the bag when collecting disposable clothing,

protective clothing and other items after use. Each packaging bag and sharps container should be attached with a label. The label should include the name of medical institution, department, date and type of waste, and mark specifically "new coronavirus infected pneumonia" or "COVID-19" in short.

(7) Process the waste from different zones. For those medical waste produced by suspected or confirmed COVID-19 patients at fever clinic and wards, before leaving the contaminated zone, the surface of the packaging bag should be sprayed uniformly and disinfected with 1000mg / L of chlorine-containing disinfectant, or a layer of medical waste packaging bag should be added on the outside. The medical waste generated in the clean zone should be disposed of according to conventional medical waste.

(8) Handle pathogen samples with care. High-risk wastes such as pathogen-containing specimens and related preservation solutions in medical waste should be pressure steam sterilized or chemically sterilized at the place of production, then collected and disposed in the same way as infectious medical waste.

(9) Central Collection and Transferring of Medical Waste

1. Management of safe transportation. Before transporting medical waste, the personnel should check whether the label and the seal of the bag or sharps container meet the requirements. While

transporting the waste, the personnel should prevent damage to the packaging bags and sharps containers filled with medical waste, avoid direct contact, leakage or spread of medical waste. Clean and disinfect the transportation tools with 1000mg / L of chlorine-containing disinfectant after the daily transportation. When the transportation tool is contaminated with infectious medical waste, it should be disinfected immediately.

2. Management of handover and storage. The temporary storage place for medical waste should be tightly closed and attended by staff, and should prevent irrelevant personnel from coming into contact with the medical waste. Medical waste should be stored in a separate and temporary area, and handed over to the medical waste disposal unit for disposal as soon as possible. The floor of temporary storage places must be disinfected with 1000mg / L of chlorine-containing disinfectant twice a day. The medical department, transport personnel, temporary storage staff, and medical waste disposal unit transfer personnel should check and register while handing over the waste, and explain to each other that it originates from patients with pneumonia or suspected patients infected with new coronavirus so that extra cautions can be taken.

3. Transfer registration. Strictly implement the joint management of hazardous waste transfer and register medical waste. The

registered content includes the source, type, weight or quantity of medical waste, handover time, final destination and signature of the manager. It must be marked specifically as COVID-19 and the registration must be kept 3 years. The medical waste disposal unit shall be notified in time for door-to-door collection or self-built medical waste disposal point, and corresponding records shall be made. Health administrations and the hospitals should strengthen their communication with the ecological environment department and medical waste disposal units in order to regulate the treatment of medical waste during the outbreak.

5.3.2 Epidemic Control Management Plan

5.3.2.1 Objective

To reduce the risk of virus transmission in the hospital, standardize the working rules of all staff including medical staff, to avoid infection.

5.3.2.2 Organization

Set up a nosocomial infection committee, composed of president, vice-presidents in charge of medical affairs, nosocomial infection, nursing and logistics, ward head nurse and ward administrative director of the hospital. The vice-president in charge of nosocomial infection leads the establishment of a nosocomial infection working group, including ward head nurses, nosocomial infection physicians, nosocomial infection nurses and logistics department liaisons who were responsible for daily nosocomial infection control.

5.3.2.3 Working plan

(1) Area division. Clearly define the contaminated area, semi-contaminated area and clean area in the hospital, and post a notice at a conspicuous location in the hospital. A prominent warning sign should be set at the junction of each district. Special entrances and exits must be arranged at the entrance and exit of the contaminated area to ensure compliance with hospital infection regulations.

(2) Carry out all staff training. Strictly abide by the system of personnel training before taking up positions. According to the nature of the position and job characteristics, determine the training content of different personnel. All personnel who need to enter the contaminated area should be given key training, proficient in the knowledge, methods and skills of the prevention and control of the disease, and raise the awareness of prevention and control. Carry out training for all workers and personnel, assist in environmental cleaning and disinfection, patient transfer, medical waste disposal, etc.

(3) Protection of medical staff and workers. On the basis of strict implementation of standard prevention, strengthen the prevention and control of contact transmission and airborne transmission. Properly select and use protective equipment and strictly implement hand hygiene.

5.3.2.4 Prevention and control system

(1) Personal protection grading system

Personal protection rating system form of Fangcang Shelter Hospital

Protection item	Primary protection	Secondary protection	Tertiary protection
Hat	*	*	*
Isolation gown	*		
Protective suit		*	*
Disposable surgical mask	*		
Medical protective mask		*	*
Goggles/protective face shield		Alternative	Both
Gloves	*	*	*
Boot/protective shoe cover		*	*

(2) Area protection grading system

Protection level form in different working areas of Fangcang Shelter Hospital

Working area/work content	Primary protection	Secondary protection	Tertiary protection
Contaminated zone		*	
Semi-contaminated zone		*	
Clean zone	*		
Specimen collection (specimens from the respiratory tract)			*
Specimen collection (specimens from the non-respiratory tract)		*	
Specimen delivery		*	
Disinfection (contaminated zone and semi-contaminated zone)		*	
Disinfection (clean zone)	*		
Patient escort and transfer		*	
Nucleic acid testing (NAT)			*
Laboratory test (specimens from the non-respiratory tract)		*	
Imaging examination		*	

(3) Donning/ Doffing PPE procedure

Standard Operating Procedure (SOP) for
Removal of Protective Suits

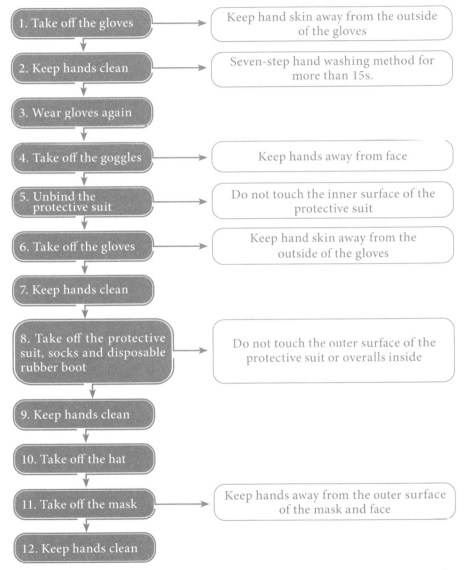

Fig. 5-7 Standard Operating Procedure for Removal of Protective Suits in the Fangcang Shelter Hospital

(4) Hygiene and disinfection of environments

Strictly implement the disinfection technical specifications of medical institutions. Clean and disinfect the diagnosis and treatment environment (air, object surface, ground, etc.), medical equipment, and patient materials. Dispose patients' respiratory secretions, excreta and vomit with care. Sterilization and cleaning appliances in contaminated areas, semi-contaminated areas, and clean areas must be marked with different colors and must not be mixed.

(5) Patient management and education

Actively carry out patient education in the hospital, and guide personal protection and cough etiquette. Masks should be worn throughout the transfer or out of the hospital for auxiliary inspections and imaging studies.

5.3.3 Security Support

5.3.3.1 Staffing

One manager in charge of providing contact information and coordinating with other departments.

5.3.3.2 Work plan

(1) Prohibit unrelated personal from entering and exiting the hospital at will.

(2) Prevent and stop riots and disputes.

(3) Coordinate and assist the transportation of supplies.

5.3.3.3 Requirement

(1) Assign at least 2 security guards at the entrance and exit of the hospital.

(2) 24 hours security patrol in the patient area.

5.3.4 Emergency Plan for Fangcang Shelter Hospital

5.3.4.1. Emergency plan for unexpected disputes

(1) Objective: Prevent the personnel from harming others out of excessive emotion; used for emergency disputes or violent incidents in sheltered hospitals.

(2) Emergency procedures.

The healthcare workers in the centers should inspect the patient and immediately report to the on-site command group if they find that the patient is prone to emotional instability. They should also coordinate with the psychological counseling staff to conduct patient counseling, and inform the security personnel to accompany the patient on site.

↓

If relevant patients do not understand these procedures and remain emotional, security guards should effectively control the situation and disperse irrelevant persons.

↓

In case of any infection or exposure during handling, appropriate disinfection and medical observation should be provided.

↓

The comprehensive group should comprehensively assess and summarize the incidents, emergency treatment and related results, and submit a summary report to the related leader.

Fig. 5-8 Emergency Response Procedure of Fangcang Shelter Hospital

5.3.4.2 Emergency plan for water or power failure

Objective: Respond to water and power failure, prevent and control water and power outage damage, ensure normal diagnosis and treatment order, ensure the safety of patients and medical personnel, and maintain the safety and stability of the hospital. Emergency procedures are as follows:

(1) Information report: When a water or power failure occurs, the first discoverer and each receiver must immediately report in accordance with the procedures and requirements of the emergency plan.

(2) Early handling: After an emergency occurs, each respondent must complete early information handling while completing the information report, or initiate an on-site emergency plan according to their responsibilities and prescribed authorities, and respond to control situations in a timely and effective manner.

(3) Emergency response: If the early treatments fail to effectively control the situation, a special emergency plan for water and power outages should be started in time. The relevant person-in-charge should direct the relevant departments to carry out the processing work. The medical treatment team leader should be responsible for directing emergency treatment. The medical staff should organize the rescue work in this area according to the on-site treatment plan for water and power failure of the department.

In addition, the emergency support of water and electricity supply should abide to the following:

(1) The members of the logistics working group should ensure smooth contact and communication at all times.

Check the water supply pipelines, circuits, and valves on a daily basis, and deal with problems in a timely manner.

(2) Train relevant logistics personnel who are required to know the emergency water supply, pipeline layout and emergency operation process.

(3) The maintenance personnel of the water and electricity should be on duty for 24 hours.

5.3.4.3 Fire incident emergency plan

Objective: To ensure the safety of personnel and property in the hospital area. In the event of a fire, avoid or mitigate casualties and property losses as much as possible. To ensure the personnel master the necessary escape skills. In case of an emergency, promptly evacuate to the nearest emergency evacuation site by using safe evacuation channels, and learn to save yourself and other people.

Emergency procedure:

(1) When a fire occurs, the person in charge on the spot should immediately arrange for the personnel in duty to use the nearest fire extinguishing equipment to extinguish the fire. During the fire extinguishing process, according to the nature of the fire (for example, when an electrical fire occurs, you must cut off the relevant

power switch of the fault location as soon as possible), and notify the security personnel to confirm the specific situation of the fire and dial 119 to call the police.

(2) Evacuate the crowd. Send evacuation instructions to the scene of the fire through emergency broadcasts. Medical staff on duty in each area should guide patients to evacuate from the fire scene in an orderly manner. The staff of the evacuation guidance group should have clear division of labor and be under unified command.

(3) Notify the medical staff resting at the nearest hotel to treat the wounded in time at the scene. Contact other neighboring hospitals for treatment if necessary.

(4) Security personnel should quickly arrive at the fire site to conduct on-site alert and maintain order.

(5) The personnel of the logistics team should register and keep the rescued and transferred materials, and cooperate with relevant departments to clean up and register fire losses.

5.3.5 Ventilation System Operation and Maintenance Support

(1) According to the division of contaminated zones, semi-contaminated zones, clean zones, medical personnel passages, and patient passages, set the operation plan. Open or close some new air

valves, supply air valves, exhaust valves, adjust the angle of some air valves, open or close air vents or windows, open or close some ventilation and air conditioning equipment.

(2) Monitor the failure alarm signals of air blower and exhaust fan at all time to ensure its normal operation. Monitor the pressure difference alarm of the air filters for all levels of the supply and exhaust system. Replace the blocked air filter in time to ensure the volume of the air supply and exhaust.

(3) The air handling unit and the new fan group should be checked regularly to keep it clean.

(4) Low-efficiency filter fan of the ventilation system should be cleaned every 2 days. Low-efficiency filter is recommended to be replaced every 1 to 2 months. Medium-efficiency filters should be checked weekly and replaced every 3 months. Sub-efficient filters should be replaced every year. If they are contaminated or blocked, they should be replaced in time. The terminal high-efficiency filter should be checked once a year, and it is recommended to replace it when the resistance exceeds the designed initial resistance of 160Pa or has been used for more than 3 years.

(5) The medium-efficiency filter in the exhaust fan group is recommended to be replaced every year. If there is pollution and blockage, it should be replaced in time.

(6) Check the return air filter regularly, and clean it once a week. If there is any special contamination, replace it in time, and wipe the inner surface of the air outlet with disinfectant.

(7) Assign special maintenance management personnel to maintain the fan following equipment instructions. Develop an operation manual for record.

(8) Operators who replace high-efficiency air filters on exhaust air must protect themselves carefully. The dismantled exhaust high-efficiency filter should be sterilized on site by professionals. The filter should be put into a safe container for sterilization, and be treated together with other medical waste.

5.4 Volunteer Service

From experiences of enlisting volunteers for previous emergency events, government should integrate social resources effectively when professional resources are inadequate and insufficient for responding to public health emergency. This includes human resources supporting the logistics services involved in Fangcang Shelter Hospitals. People who register as volunteers must meet the relevant criteria and requirements. Most importantly, they should volunteer under their freewill and expect no economic return.

5.4.1 Criteria and Requirement

(1) Strictly follow the staff arrangements and schedules set by Control Team when participating in volunteer events.

(2) Volunteers in Shelter Hospitals must have good health conditions and wear PPE when participating in relevant work. They should be trained before starting volunteer work. Volunteers should stay in their own work zone. Cross-zone working is strictly prohibited.

(3) When recruiting volunteers, priorities should be given to people with medical or psychological education background. Volunteers should also be familiar with epidemic control and prevention campaigns, relevant policies and regulations, and knowledge and theories relating to psychological interventions.

(4) When giving services, volunteers should always apply the principle of "safety-first". Regular education and training on epidemic control and prevention should be given in a timely manner. Strictly monitor and supervise on proper PPE donning procedure. Approaching work without wearing the PPE is prohibited. Volunteers who fail to meet the training expectation are not allowed to approach their work. Reasonable job division and schedules should be implemented. Closely monitor on the number and shift time of volunteers.

5.4.2 Job Division Scheme

Professional Medical Assistant: Volunteers need to enter high-risk contaminated zone, to assist medical staff in daily check on patients.

Medical Supplies Logistics: Deliver medical supplies including medicine, equipment and facilities and PPE to assigned areas. Volunteers are also responsible for organizing and recording the medical supplies.

Living Engagement Support: Volunteers are responsible for providing social and living support for patients and medical staff. This includes transportation, food supplies, and other living engagement supports. Meanwhile, volunteers should be responsible for the maintenance of the power, water and heating supplies.

5.4.3 Job Design

(1) Professional Medical Assistant: The main job content is to maintain the public order in Fangcang Shelter Hospitals, as well as control the medical supplies in urgent need, and organize the information of admitted patients. Take Zall (Wuhan Salon) Fangcang Shelter Hospitals as an example, there are 54 volunteers who are responsible for cleaning and disinfection of the equipment and facilities. There are three shifts per day, and they work 24/7 to disinfect and dispose the medical waste.

(2) Medical Supplies Logistics: The main responsibility is to transport, deliver and organize various catalog of medical supplies, which include medicine, PPEs, respirators, surgery masks and gloves.

(3) Living Engagement Support: The main responsibility is to ensure the essential living and social engagement activities of medical staff and patients. This includes the diary plan, transportation and other engagement support related to culture and social engagement. Meanwhile, they also take the responsibility of maintaining and monitoring on the power, water and heat supplies in the hospitals, in order to respond to emergency events in a timely manner. Take Zall (Wuhan Salon) Fangcang Shelter Hospitals as an example, there were approximately 100 volunteers participating in the reconstruction of the hospitals and they completed the redevelopment within 72 hours. They set up a reading corner, power charging center, food and beverage center, entertainment center and other functional room. Moreover, they ensured the distribution of supplies, which were donated by public community. They also monitored the condition of power, water and heating system, to prevent any malfunction and breakdown.

References

[1] Chen Simiao, Zhang Zongjiu, Yang Juntao, et al. Fangcang Shelter Hospitals: A Novel Concept for Responding to Public Health Emergencies [J]. The Lancet, 2020.

[2] Medical Administration and Hospital Authority of National Health Committee of the PRC, Medical Management and Service Guidance Center of National Health Committee of the PRC. Work Manual for Fangcang Shelter Hospital (3rd Edition) [S]. 2020.

[3] Department of Housing and Urban-Rural Development of Zhejiang Province. Technical Guidelines for Centralized Receiving and Treatment in Fangcang Shelter Hospital (Trial) [S]. 2020.

[4] Department of Housing and Urban-Rural Development of Hubei Province. Technical Requirements for Design and Reconstruction of Fangcang Shelter Hospital (Revised Edition) [S]. 2020.

[5] General Office of Ministry of Housing and Urban-Rural Development of the PRC, General Office of National Health Committee of the PRC. Guidelines for Design of Emergency Treatment Facilities in COVID-19 (Trial) [S]. 2020.

[6] Gu Ming, Hua Xiaoli, Chen Jun, Zeng Fang, Zhou Tao, Zhang Yu, Shi Chen. Pharmacy Administration and Pharmaceutical Care Practice in Jianghan Fangcang Shelter Hospital [J]. China Pharmacist, 2020, 23 (04):702-706.

Acknowledgments

Jack Ma Foundation

Alibaba Foundation

China First Metallurgical Group Co., Ltd.

CITIC General Institute of Architectural Design
and Research Co., Ltd.

Department of Housing and Urban-Rural Development
of Hubei Province

Department of Housing and Urban-Rural Development
of Zhejiang Province

Central South Architectural Design Institute Co., Ltd.

Wuhan Real Estate Group Co., Ltd.

Wuhan Hanyang Municipal Construction Group Co., Ltd.

Hubei Yangtze River Industrial Investment Group Co., Ltd.

Wuhan Shooting School

Zall Foundation is a public welfare organization established in Wuhan, Hubei Province, China. Founded by Yan Zhi, Chairman of Zall Holdings Company Limited, the foundation mainly focuses on public welfare activities such as disaster relief, poverty alleviation, student assistance, culture and sport events, and ecological and environmental protection.

After the outbreak of the novel coronavirus disease in 2020, Zall Foundation greatly relieved the pressure of the medical system in Hubei by quickly launching various assistance. They donated a large number of urgently needed medical protection equipment to Hubei for fighting against epidemic; provided materials to renovate existing hospitals into emergency hospitals to treat suspected and confirmed COVID-19 patients; converted public venues to Fangcang Shelter Hospitals to treat patients with mild to moderate symptoms of COVID-19; and offered logistic support to guarantee the smooth operation of these hospitals.

In addition, Zall Foundation actively participates in global fight against COVID-19 by donating medical supplies to 16 countries. It continues to share its experiences by publishing the timely books, *Fangcang Shelter Hospitals for COVID-19: Construction and Operation Manual*, and *Emergency Hospitals for COVID-19: Construction and Operation Manual*. Currently, these two booklets have been translated into more than 20 languages.

Fangcang Shelter Hospitals for COVID-19: Construction and Operation Manual

Editor-in-Chief: Yan Zhi
Editors: Zhang Liang, Du Shuwei, Fang Li, Pan Zijing, Cheng Longhua
Translator: Yan Ge
English Proofreader: Wang Sida
Layout Designers: Huang Xuan, Song Jie, Ye Qinyun